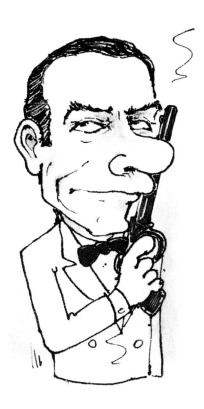

SHUPREME SHEX·GOD
OF SHCOTLAND:
SIR SEAN CONNERY

ERRATUM

Chapter 5: for *porn* read *prawn*

The Cannae Sutra

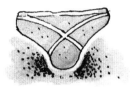

contains nuts

THE SCOTS 'JOY OF SEX'!

THE CANNAE SUTRA

RUPERT BESLEY

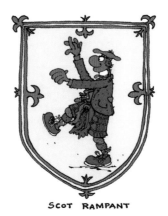

SCOT RAMPANT

BIRLINN

ACKNOWLEDGEMENTS

With many thanks for their considerable contributions and support
to Hugh Andrew, Lindsey and Marcus Besley, Laura Esselmont,
Aline Hill, Jim Hutcheson, Andrew Simmons and others.

Material (carefully selected!) from the Get by in Gaelic section
is reproduced by kind permission of Morag MacNeill from
her book *Everyday Gaelic*.

First published in 2006 by
Birlinn Limited
West Newington House
10 Newington Road
Edinburgh EH9 1QS

www.birlinn.co.uk
Reprinted 2007
Text and illustrations copyright © Rupert Besley 2006

ISBN10: 1 84158 484 3
ISBN13: 978 1 84158 484 3

British Library Cataloguing-in-Publication Data
A catalogue record for this book is available from
the British Library

Designed and typeset by Robbie Porteous
Printed and bound in Poland

Contents

1. Preface

SEX IN EDINBURGH, as everyone knows, is what the coal comes in. It's tea-time in Morningside. It's the instrument played by Charlie Parker. It's something they do down south; it's not what's done in Scotland. Having sex is what happens four times a year, when the coalman delivers.

But there is more to Scotland than meets the aye. Scots have always been fond of their oats. Sex and Scotland may seem unlikely bed-fellows, but beneath the covers there is much to explore. Settle down somewhere comfortable. Loosen that straitjacket. And now read on.

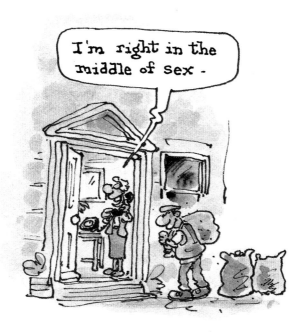

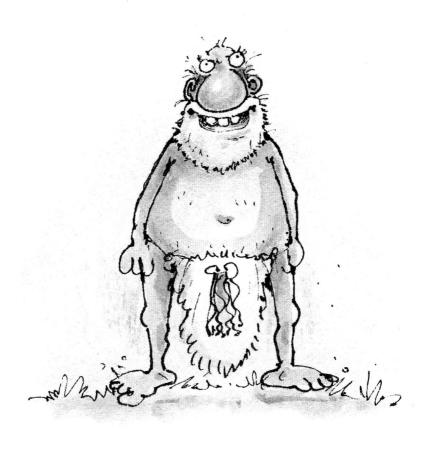

OUR FOREBEARS . . .

2. From the Beginning

SEX IN SCOTLAND was first discovered by Edinburgh-born Marie Stopes in the early part of the twentieth century. It was a discovery that upset a lot of people, including her husband Reginald. (Their marriage was annulled in 1916 after five years, on grounds of non-consummation.) Another to be rattled was Walter Blackie, the Glasgow publisher. As he put it to Marie Stopes when rejecting her manuscript for *Married Love*, 'I think there's far too much talking and writing about these things already.'

Twenty-five years on, Mr J.F. Coates, member for New South Wales, told the Australian Parliament, 'The Empire today has three enemies – all from Munich. One is Hitler, the other Goebbels and the third that doctor of German philosophy and science - Dr Marie Stopes. The greatest of these is Marie Stopes.'

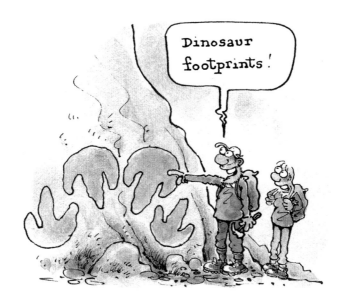

Stopes did not invent sex. She was just among the first to stop pretending it didn't exist. With her PhD from Munich in palaeobotany, Dr Stopes would have known that sex has been knocking around an awful long time. Even in Scotland.

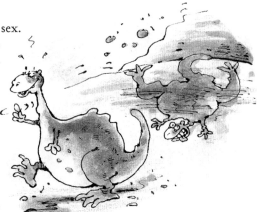

Early life-forms multiplied by simple fission. But breaking up is hard to do. Ever since the first speck of protozoa got the hots for its neighbour, sex has been the driving force of all that followed. That at least was how, through steamed-up glasses, Freud saw it.

At first all went swimmingly. Then along came the dinosaurs, rarely able to get their act together – so they died out.

The animal kingdom had another 60-odd million years in which to develop and refine the arts of sexual encounter to the level enjoyed by Stone-Age Man and little changed since.

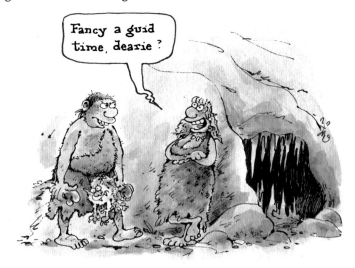

THE OLDEST PROFESSION

PICTS, ROMANS AND NORSEMEN

CRUITHNE, SON OF CINGI, the father of the Picts, reigned for a hundred years. He had seven sons: Cat, Ce, Circinn, Fortran, Fotlaig, Fidach – and Fib.

The Picts were a hardy race, who wore no clothes, but painted themselves blue instead. They spent their time huddled over hot drinks in the Highlands, leaving cup and ring marks on every flat surface in Alba. Recent researches have cast doubt on these facts: Pictish carvings do show figures wearing clothes, as may also have been the case with some of the elephants, mermaids and serpents that lived alongside. Pictish inscriptions are in ogham, a system of lines and bars intelligible only at supermarket checkouts.

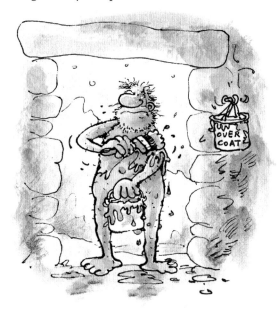

TRADITIONAL UNDERSTANDING OF PICT GETTING DRESSED IN THE MORNING

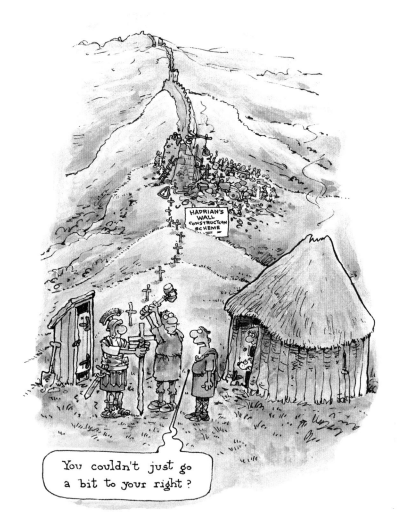

Don't be fooled by the colosseum at Oban: the Romans were not a great success in the north. A few brave souls made it past Hadrian's Wall to Falkirk. Here they put up another wall, 37 miles long but mainly of grass. A 12-foot high mound of turf was never going to halt marauding Picts in their tracks. Homesick and lovesick, with their fashionable outfits fast losing shape in the rain, the Romans retreated

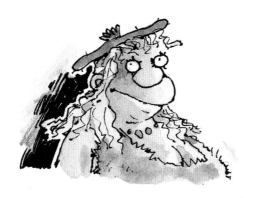

SEX·SIRENS OF SCOTLAND :
Stone-Age Times

to Glasgow and Edinburgh, where they cleaned up in the ice-cream business instead.

Little is known about what went on in the Dark Ages. All we have is a few names and dates of early kings and sub-kings, from Fergus MacErc to Lulach the Fool. The House of Alpin and its immediate successors stuck mostly with Kenneths and Malcolms and Constantines, with the odd throat-clearing Aedh, Eochaid, Giric and Duff thrown in for good measure. The Vikings did a better line in names. They had earls of Orkney called Thorfinn Raven-Feeder and Sigurd the Stout.

Rolf the Goer

William the Lyon (1143–1214, married to Ermengarde) was the man who brought the rearing lion into Scotland's royal coat of arms, along with the motto, 'Nemo me impune lacessit' ('No one gets away with calling me puny' or 'Wha daur meddle wi' me?'). Replacing the earlier emblem (a boar) meant a trawl through the royal menagerie, and ended in a toss-up between rampant lion and rampant gerbil; the lion won.

The first signs of sexual awakening in Scotland date back to the medieval era, when days were cold and knights were bold. The religious houses (Ardchattan, Sweetheart, Nunraw) were among the first to get a name for such things.

It's the same every Christmas – all the novices get drunk at the party and then do rude things round the copier!

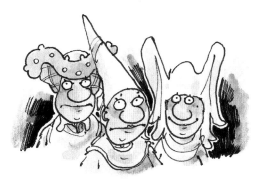

SEX SIRENS OF SCOTLAND:
Medieval Sugababes.

Medieval interlude:
The Hamecumming

A SCOTTISH PLAY, 1292

DRAMATIS PERSONAE:
The MacBoghead of MacBoghead
Muckle Meg, Lady MacBoghead
Alastair Campbell, a Messenger
Ladies of the Chamber
Assorted pages, swains and other faeries
Dogberry and Tytchemarsh, gardeners of Glen Boghead
Henbane, Toadspit and Spleen, three witches.

Act 1. Sc 1. *Dark chamber below the Castle of Boghead. Witches dance round cauldron, engaged in trad preparation of haggis.*

1ST WITCH:	Eye of newt, half tongue of frog,
	Flav'ring, aspartame, phlegm of dog.
2ND W:	Stir ingredients with a broom –
	Ah, that rhymes with gloom and doom.

Act 1. Sc 2. *Upstairs, Lady MacBoghead's bedchamber. Fair maids by window spinning, reading, doing Sudoku. Gallery minstrels, Big Mac and his Rumble Tum Ceilidh Band, play popular dance tunes. Lady MacB paces by fireside.*

Suddenly, a great clang below, followed by approaching squeaks and clanks, echoing eerily up the spiral staircase. All look up.

FAIR MAID: Crivens, maistress, 'tis the laird,
               Hame fra' the whaurs just as ye feared–

Lady MacB throws Fair Maid a thunderous look.

FM: Nae, 'whaurs', ye ken, just as in fighting,
               Not 'whores', the ladies, oft inviting.

LADY MACB: (*suddenly, with expansive gesture to all the merrymakers*)
               Be aff, git oot, awa' the noo
               Hide all things festive, quickly, shoo
               Begone, young fiddler, fast make haste,
               Else Laird will beat me – to a paste.

Door swings open. Enter, awkwardly, a figure all in armour.

MACB: Thingle blear garp goodrie bloo
               Thang gogginge fylfot scoudrie noo
LADY MACB: I canny staun a word ye say.
               Fust up, yon visor must away.
MACB: (*gesturing downwards*)
               Skrark gargle flubbit John o' Groats
               Blurk dongle fanging blathered scrote–
LADY MACB: Four lang years without being naughty,
               Haste, varmint, fetch ye WD 40.

Exit Marr, a dog-eared page. Large maidens with poker and firebrace lever up visor on helmet.

LADY MACB: So –
MACB: 'Tis me –
LADY MACB: And how thy journey?
MACB: Ach, nose to tail until the border,
               Then better stretch as far as Lauder,
               But next, alas, what fule I am,
               By Callander the usual jam–

LADY MACB: 'Tis not the route that I'd ha' taken—
MACB: Hush, Meg, within me feelings waken.
                For travel info I'm not back.
                I need my oats. That's what I lack.
                Unhose me, ma'am. Prepare thy bed.
LADY MACB: (*grappling with rusted fixings*)
                Less easy done, so easy said.
                Rerebrace, tassets, byrnie, I wist
                All of them rusted by dree Scottish mist.
MACB (*angry*)
                Rusted, crusted, busted – fie!

In sudden rage, brings iron gauntlet crashing down on trestle table by window, causing small key to bounce out of previously covered goblet and drop into moat below.

LADY MACB: (*reproachful*)
                So that is where yon key was hid,
                For chastitie belt, beneath that lid.
                And now 'tis gone, well, thanks a lot
                My hips are sealed, thou plookie faced clot.
                Undone am I, yet not undone –
                So much for ovens and a bun.

Curtain falls. End of Act One.

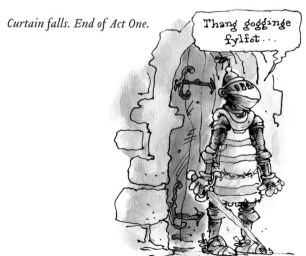

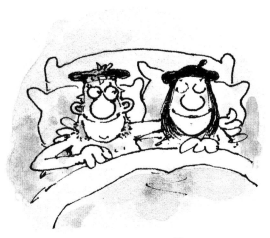

och la la

THE AULD ALLIANCE

THE AULD ALLIANCE was signed in 1295, but Norman/Norseman links go back a good deal further. Torf Einar, Earl of Orkney in 910, was brother of Hrolf, who grabbed what then became Normandy. Hrolf (or Rollo) was also known as Rolf the Ganger (or, in some translations, Rolf the Goer). He was said to have had legs so long that, as he swept down on horseback from the north, he appeared to be walking. Not bad, even on a Shetland pony.

As long the English have been around being English, Scots and French have joined forces against the common foe. The down side of this for Scotland was the number of mercenaries slaughtered in the Hundred Years War. (Joan of Arc had her Scottish Guard – no record, though, of the Scottish Guard ever having had Joan of Arc.) The good news was that for several centuries the wine importers of Leith had first choice of all the best French clarets, leaving the English to gag on the dregs.

Some took the alliance a bit too literally. In 1563 Pierre de Chastelard, lovesick French poet, was found hiding under the bed of Mary, Queen of Scots in Rossend Castle, Burntisland. As it was a second offence, he was dragged out, tried and hanged next day in front of the queen, crying out, 'Adieu, most beautiful and most cruel princess in the world!'

Another casualty of the Auld Alliance was Kenneth Mackenzie, the Brahan Seer. The seventeenth-century Mackenzie (aka Coinneach Odhar) is credited with predicting trains, television, North Sea oil, the Caledonian Canal, the Battle of Culloden, World War Two (but not One?), the collapse of Fearn Abbey, the Scottish Parliament and the Channel Tunnel, but nothing on Scotland's performance in any World Cup. In the end he saw – or said – rather more than was good for him. When Isabella, Countess of Seaforth, and not one of Nature's greatest beauties, asked the seer why her husband was still not back from Paris, Mackenzie hesitated to reply. Pressed for an answer, he said (correctly, as it turned out) that the Earl of Seaforth was dallying with 'one fairer than yourself'. Sparks flew and Mackenzie went on to predict, again with unerring accuracy, the end of the line of Seaforth (a deaf and dumb earl, fathering four sons, who would predecease him, and two daughters, one of whom would kill the other. In 1823 the pony carriage driven by Lady Hood spilled over, killing her sister, Lady Caroline Mackenzie, second daughter of the last Lord Seaforth.) Mackenzie was rewarded for this by being stuffed head first into a barrel of boiling tar and left at Chanonry Point in the Moray Firth. That he hadn't foreseen.

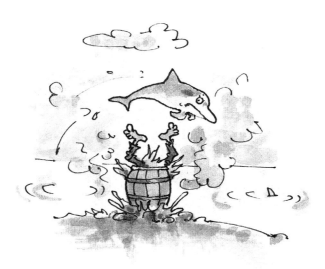

BEDROOM SCENES

FEW MONARCHS ever found love quite so romantically as did James I of Scotland. With his family at each other's throats in 1406, the young James Stewart spent a miserable month in hiding on the Bass Rock, awaiting shipment to safety in France. But his unkind uncle, the Duke of Albany, got word of this move and passed it on to the English. The eleven-year-old prince was duly intercepted off Flamborough Head and held captive in England for eighteen years, while Albany, as regent, declined to cough up the ransom.

Cooped up and pining, the royal prisoner stared long from his window. One day (or several days – she was determined to catch his eye) he spotted the comely form of Joanna Beaufort, cousin of Henry IV, walking her dog in the garden below. He chucked her a rose and she wore it next day. Love blossomed, as did the romantic verse he wrote her (all without spellchecker) –

> *. . . And there-with kest I doun myn eye ageyne,*
> *Quhare as I sawe, walking under the toure,*
> *Full secretly, new cummyn hir to pleyne,*
> *The fairest or the freschest yonge floure*
> *That ever I sawe, me thoght, before that houre,*
> *For quhich sodayn abate, anon astert*
> *The blude of all my body to my hert . . .*

The two were married in Southwark Cathedral. With promises to pay an extortionate ransom and not to attack the English rear, James and Joanna were finally free to leave for Scotland. Thirteen years later, their lives together ended in circumstances far from romantic.

In the private apartment of the Perth friary where they had sought refuge, James I was hacked to death in front of his wife. It was a revenge killing by Scottish nobles. Hearing his attackers approach, James tore up a floorboard, hoping to escape down the sewer beneath. But he himself had had the other end of the drain blocked up just three days earlier, as tennis balls kept disappearing down it. At the sound of commotion coming up the stairs, the Queen's lady-in-waiting rushed to bar the bedroom door – but the bolt was missing. Thrusting her arm through the brackets, Catherine Douglas gained for her king a few seconds more of life and, for herself, a broken arm and the name thenceforth of Katy Bar-lass.

JAMES, JAMES

THE BEDROOM ACTIVITIES of James IV and James V left Scotland well stocked with little bastards – the latter is reckoned to have fathered at least seven James Stewarts, each by different mothers. Held virtual prisoner in Stirling Castle, the young King James V gained a worthy reputation for slipping out in disguise each evening to visit his subjects and learn of their lives. It was the subjects with daughters that he visited most and the abbeys of Scotland filled up with their offspring. According to John Knox, some dispraised James 'for the defoulling of menis wyffes and virgines'.

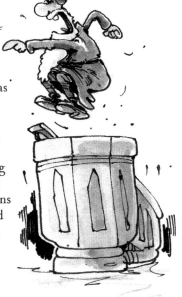

James IV, meanwhile, had played the field, both before and after his unhappy marriage to Margaret Tudor, who was no pin-up. The Marriage of Thistle and Rose was never a comfortable union. Instead, James had various children by different mistresses, chief among them Lady Kennedy, also known as Flaming Janet. All this he managed while continuing to wear about his loins the harness chain he had donned as penance for his father's death and vowed to keep on till his dying day. On the eve of Flodden, James visited Lady Heron in her castle. She had difficulties with the chain in bed and persuaded him to remove it. The rest is history.

JOHN KNOX SHARING HIS THOUGHTS ON WOMEN

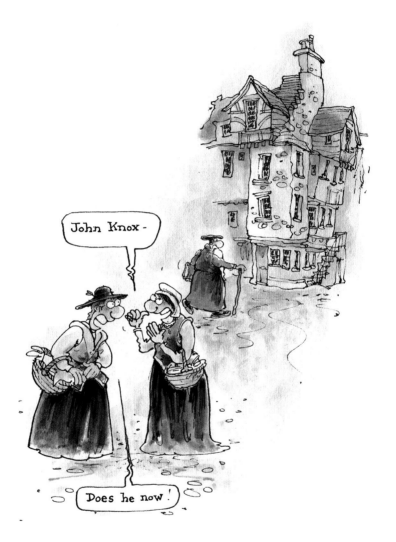

ROUGH WOOINGS

AS PART OF his cunning plan for world domination, Henry VIII decided his young son Edward should marry the similarly young Mary, Queen of Scots. But her mother had other ideas. Not to be beaten, Henry prepared to send an army – and navy – north. Such things rarely go to plan; first of all, Henry died. Protector Somerset took over, but, far from being able to wrap the Scots around his little finger, he found 36,000 armed men lined up to meet him on Musselburgh golf course. Ten thousand Scots are said to have died on Black Saturday, including some unlucky enough to be flattened by cannonballs from the warships parked out in the Firth of Forth. The Battle of Pinkie was an English victory, but not much of one. The reign of terror that followed was enough to unite Scots against English occupation forever (or at least till holiday homes came in). Mary was hustled out of Scotland to marry the heir to France instead. Somerset fell from power and was executed for treason in 1552. That's what comes of trying to force affections upon another.

MARY, QUEEN OF SCOTS

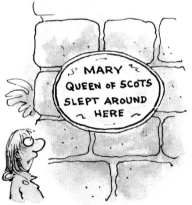

QUEEN OF SCOTLAND at six days old, Mary married the dauphin in 1558. He became king of France the following year and the year after that he was dead. Back in Scotland, Mary nursed her cousin, Lord Darnley, through measles and married him. It was a rash decision. Within a year they had fallen out. Darnley led the gang which burst into the royal apartments to murder Rizzio, Mary's favoured Italian secretary, before her eyes. (The spot on the floor in Holyroodhouse boasts a ghostly stain, which returns each time it is removed – even with Jif.) A year later, Darnley's house was blown up and his strangled syphilitic body found out in the garden, along with that of his crumpled page.

Chief suspect was the Earl of Bothwell. Mary married Bothwell. They parted, being forced to flee Scotland in different directions. Mary was held prisoner in England for nineteen years before she was executed in 1587.

When Mary left Scotland, her half-brother, Moray, took over as regent; two years later he was shot dead in Linlithgow. Next up was the Earl of Lennox, father of Darnley; he took charge for a year, before being killed at Stirling. The Earl of Mar, who followed as regent, died within a year, allegedly poisoned by Morton. The next regent was Morton, who six years later was executed on The Maiden, the early form of guillotine that he himself had introduced to Scotland as a way of being tough on crime, tough on the causes of crime. Mary, Queen of Scots, is agreed by all to be the Most Romantic Figure in Scottish History.

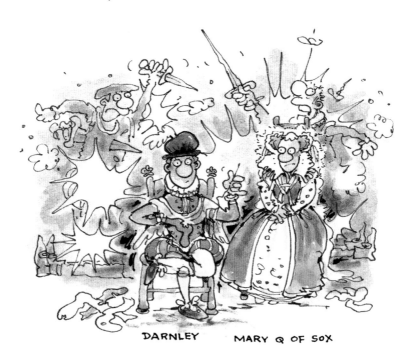

DARNLEY   MARY Q OF SOX

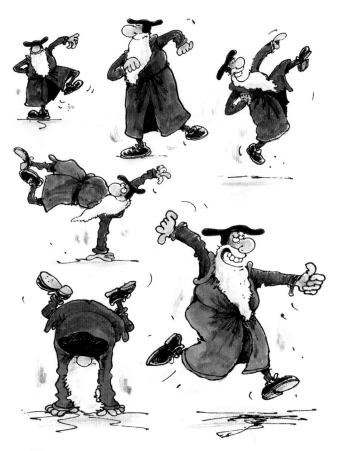

JOHN KNOX ON THE DANCE FLOOR

OPPORTUNITY KNOX

NOT THE GRIM Calvinist of popular legend, John Knox was a man of passion, full of big surprises. After the death of his first wife, Knox married a girl of seventeen, who bore him three daughters; he was three times her age. As an elderly preacher and in failing health, Knox was still described as 'so active and vigorous that he was like to ding that pulpit in blads and flee out of it'. He now lies buried under space 23 of the visitors' car park by the Cathedral of St Giles.

THE YOUNG PRETENDER AND ENLIGHTENMENT

IN 1745, for one fine month of high hopes and big balls, Bonnie Prince Charlie reigned in Edinburgh. But it was all a dream and not to be. After Culloden, the government of England set about the obliteration of Scotland. The Disarming Act was used to get rid of

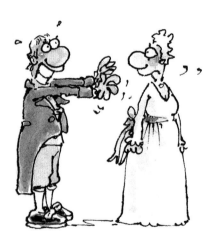

Henry Mackenzie
'The Man of Feeling'

the deadliest weapons of the Scots, beginning with the kilt. Tartan, clans and shortbread were down to follow. As ever with government policies, what happened next was the opposite of what was intended. Scotland hit a Golden Age (tarnished somewhat by the Clearances). Edinburgh erupted with poets and painters, writers, philosophers and bores: Hume, Smith, Scott, Burns, Hogg, Raeburn, Ramsay... all the way down to Henry Mackenzie, the Man of Feeling. Far from disbanding, new regiments of kilted Highlanders were formed, much in demand with the English government to fight its battles of imperial conquest around the world. Suddenly all were keen – even the King – to establish their Scottish credentials and seek out the new traditional tartan they were entitled to wear. Two centuries on, Scottish ancestry is huge business, enabling countless millions across five continents to prove their descent from Flora MacDonald.

ROMANTIC ERA IN SCOTLAND

The Ploughman-Poet Enters Edinburgh Society

Sc. 1. *Lord Monboddo's Salon, Edinburgh. 1786.*
Room filled with philosophers, swots, sycophants, society ladies, eighteenth-century celebs and the clink of teacups. Hair-clippings on floor.

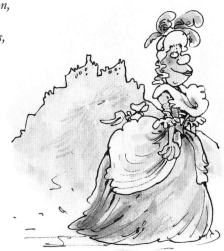

CORDELIA, LADY COWDENBEATH:
Don't you think it demp for the time of ye-ah?
MACASKILL OF THAT ILK:
Permit me to point out, ma'am, that is but the consequence of a seasonal low moving up from the Azores.

SEX-SIRENS OF SCOTLAND: the 18th century

LADY C: And allow me to respond, kind sirrah, thet in metters meteorological you are most frightfully well informed–
MACA (*beaming*): Dark outside it may be, but this is the Age of Enlightenment.

A polite ripple of applause goes round the room. Boswell whips out his notebook.

LORD SUCCUP: Well faid, fir, if I may fay fo.

Sudden commotion outside. All rush to windows to observe strange coach pull up outside and occupant step down (from two-wheeled cab with spoiler, go-faster stripes, fluffy dice and chromium gig-lamps, drawn by loudly farting carthorse).

LADY GOLSPIE: Hansom, eh?
COUNTESS OF CUMBERNAULD: Nae kidding, ratface.
JEREMIAH CLARKSON: Correction, ladies, that is the new Cartina, with 2.1 inch twin-valve sprocket flange and side-impact halter noose –

Enter R. Burns, mud-caked and dishevelled.

LADY C: Would you laike a cup of tay?
BURNS: Whitthebollockecclefechangobshite–

Ladies swoon. The Earl of Troon bursts into tears. Servants rush in with pomanders, smelling salts and little packs of pot-pourri, reduced since Christmas, from the Hoose of Fraser.

LADY C: Was thet one lump or two?

SC. 2. *Next morning, in the bed of Lady Cowdenbeath.*

LADY C: (*crimson in face from exertions*) And still it rains –
BURNS: O, my Luve's like a red, red rose . . .

MUCH DEBATED IN literary circles is what went on at the Riddell's one evening in 1793. The exact details will never be known, but, from his abject letter of apology sent next day, it would appear that Burns disgraced himself and drink was to blame. After the ladies had withdrawn from the dinner table, the men were left talking about the Rape of the Sabine Women. Rejoining company in the drawing-room, they then staged an all too realistic enactment of the subject under discussion. Mrs Riddell was not amused.

In the words so frequently sung:

Should auld acquaintance be forgot
And ever brought to mind?
Should wotsit doo-dah be tra-lah
Lah lah lah auld lang syne?
Lah lah-la thingummy hoojit
Doo-dah doo-dah doo-dah-do
Dee-dum a cup o' kindness yet
For the sake of auld lang syne.

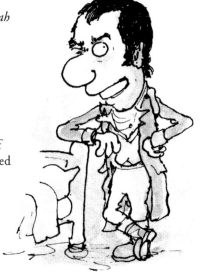

Robert Burns was judged
All-Time Greatest Scot (poll of
academics and historians carried
out by *Scotland On Sunday*) –
ahead of St Columba and
Jock Stein.

SEX·GODS OF SCOTLAND:
ROBERT BURNS
(who fathered 13 children
by 5 women including
9 by his wife)

BONNIE PRINCE GEORGIE

IN A TARTANFEST stage-managed by Sir Walter Scott, George IV paid a royal visit to Edinburgh for 'one and twenty daft days' in 1822. The monarch caused much merriment by donning a kilt – over pink silk stockings. Passing through Leith, George IV declared its fishwives the handsomest women he ever had seen – that from one who had seen a few.

As a young prince, George got involved first with the actress Perdita Robinson. After a sticky relationship with Lady Melbourne, he entered into secret marriage with Mrs Maria Fitzherbert. In between, he managed to get through a good deal of bedding material, claiming from each conquest a lock of hair as keepsake. By the end of his reign there were said to be seven thousand such envelopes containing his treasures. He died of exhaustion.

There was one person not much impressed by the Prince Regent in bed and that was his first cousin, Caroline of Brunswick-Wolfenbuttel, whom he married officially. The two soon discovered they had much in common: revulsion for each other. The Prince Regent spent the first night of his honeymoon drunk in the fireplace, which suited them both. For his coronation twenty-five years later, George IV made meticulous plans to keep his wife out of the ceremony. Egged on by the crowd outside, Caroline hammered on the abbey doors, but prize-fighters had been hired as pages and her way was barred.

BALMORALITY

AT BALMORAL, court protocol was followed with all the strictness customary in royal residences. In sexual activity, as with speaking, sitting down or starting to eat, it was necessary for the Queen to start first. For many a long August week, house-guests on the royal estates would pace, white-faced and tetchy, awaiting the signal (the raising of a rooftop flag by day or firing of a maroon at night). Footmen and valets would then be sent hurrying down corridors with small cards on silver salvers and the entire building would start to shake, from basement to turret, for maybe thirty seconds or more, until the sounding of a gong and restoration of funereal quiet. This was a practice which, touchingly, Victoria insisted should continue after the sad passing of Albert.

The long years of widowhood were lean times for royalty with urges. While a desolate Victoria sought comfort in the company of her faithful servant, Billy Connolly, other members of her large family were hard-pressed to keep a stiff upper lip. Opportunities for liaison were generally limited to a quick grope in the back row of the house-party photograph or a tumble in the laundry-cupboard with a minor duchess in the later rounds of a game of Sardines.

The ban on fun and frolics hit all ranks of society between Braemar and Ballater, with two notable exceptions. Victoria herself struck lucky, out stalking on the hills. Little matter that John Brown was of lowly status, rough tongued and had red knees; their eyes met across a crowded

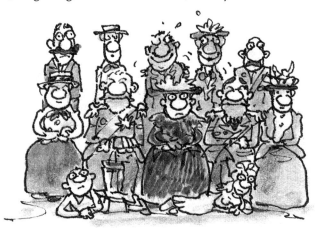

moor and two hearts beat as one. Rumours spread about the ghillie (whose royal duties included mounting Queen Victoria), but, in the absence of mobile phones, nothing was ever proved.

The other personage to escape the clampdown was the Prince of Wales (who turned into Edward VII). Thanks to the presence of Mrs Keppel along the Tweed, railway timetables in Scotland were thrown to the winds, royal trains commissioned and new track laid – all for a Bertie weekend in Berwick.

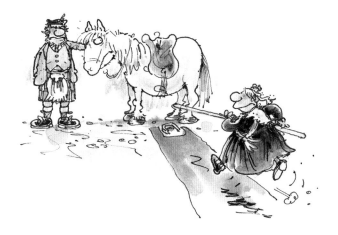

When he became king, Edward was hailed as 'the monarch to make things hum'. The old way of life, little altered for two thousand years, came to an end in the twentieth century, thanks to the arrival of cars, television, rubber wotsits and computers. In Scotland the century saw massive changes. In came flared trousers, plastic cabers and the self-untying shoelace. Among the first exponents of this flash new age were the American servicemen posted north in wartime. The GIs brought with them glamour and style, chewing-gum and nylons (snapped up for midge hoods). And then there were the Sixties. When Victoria's long reign drew to a close in Scotland (around 1969), the time was right for revolution. Love was in the air. It was the era of sexual liberation and everything changed. Except on Lewis.

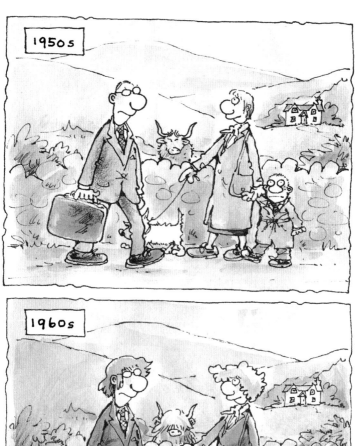

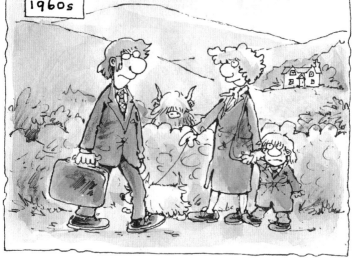

THE SEXUAL REVOLUTION IN SCOTLAND (BEFORE/AFTER)

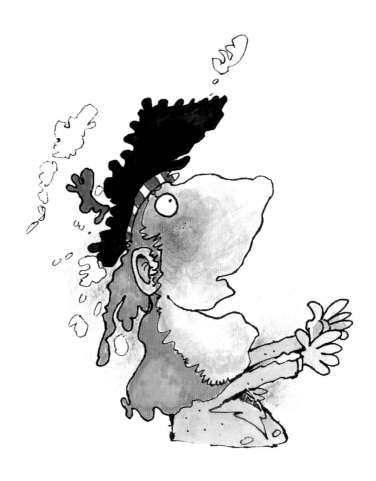

3. Outlying Parts

MENTION SCOTLAND AND people generally think first of the Highlands. In fact, most Scots live abroad, in Canada, America, Australia and Surrey.

Scotland itself can be divided into two parts, Highlands and Lowlands. The Highlands can be divided into two parts, Highlands and Islands. The Islands can be divided into two parts, Northern and Western. The Lowlands are just the Lowlands. This is where Scots are generally to be found, other parts having been taken over by English people who have fled north – to escape the domination of Scots in Westminster.

East Coast Scots tend to face west, away from the prevailing wind. West Coast Scots tend to face east, for similar reasons. With their diverse ethnic origins, Scots are proud of their regional differences. No two Scots are ever quite the same, though laboratories south of Edinburgh are working on the problem. Any generalisation about Scots is bound to be inaccurate, including this one, but fun to make all the same.

GRETNA GREEN

GATEWAY TO SCOTLAND and Caribbean of its day. It was north to Gretna that generations of love's young tearaways came, if they needed to get married in a hurry and/or without the consent of parents (required in England from 1754 for anyone under twenty-one). A note in the toast-rack, a fumble in the bus station and, several million miles later (unless coming from Carlisle), the knot was tied. Gretna claims to be the most famous marriage venue in the world and the wedding place of many a well-known couple, including Robin Hood and Maid Marian (and no doubt Tristan and Isolde too). Laws have changed, but Gretna is still the place where more than a thousand couples choose to get hitched each year, performing their marital duties over the blacksmith's anvil.

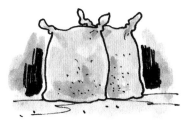

STRAIGHT SEX

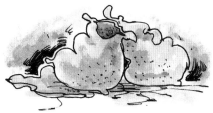

CASUAL SEX

A fun-loving guy from Tahiti
Fell foul of his Dumfriesshire sweetie;
When he removed her top layer
She replied with a glare,
'That's not what we do in Dalbeattie!'

EDINBURGH

EDINBURGH IS FAMOUS for its passages and entries. Sex takes place in Edinburgh throughout the month of August, when thousands flock into the city to perform. Each year the Festival attracts a huge crowd of thespians who meet up in worn sleeping-bags on cold floors to do their bit for the spread of culture. Edinburgh was recently voted fifth most-talked-about city in the world and ranked fourteenth overall out of the Top Fifty list of most glamorous and interesting cities. (Birmingham came in forty-fifth and Belfast forty-sixth, but ahead of Beirut.) Edinburgh folk value fidelity – hence the statue to Greyfriars Bobby, the small dog that stayed by his master's grave for fourteen years (the pie-shop alongside was just a coincidence).

GLASGOW

IF EDINBURGH FOLK have a reputation for being somewhat buttoned-up over sex, Glaswegians are quite the reverse, letting it all hang out. The city even provides small shelters along main roads for purposes of sex. These are positioned at regular intervals and can easily be accessed by bus. (Booking advisable at weekends.) Gay venues are to be found north of Glasgow, on the Campsie Fells. Alongside Goa and an island of Hawaii, Glasgow was newly voted holiday hotspot by Frommer's Travel Guides. Scotland's second city was the only place in Western Europe to make it into the Top Ten of trendy destinations.

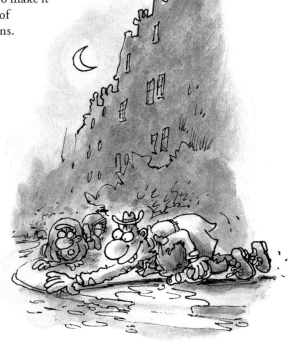

KERB - CRAWLING
IN GLASGOW

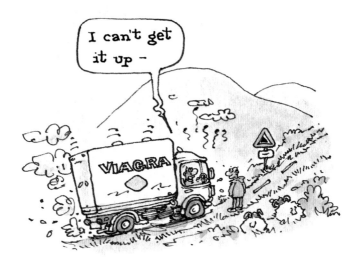

THE WEST COAST

THE WEST COAST of Scotland is a maze of islands and peninsulas of incomparable beauty. Access has never been easy in these parts. Down the water from Glasgow are the Kyles of Bute, where in former times Highland cattle heading south were required to swim the narrows as best they could (few ever mastered butterfly or backstroke). These days a car ferry makes the crossing, enabling them to drive over instead. CalMac ferries are part of the way of life here; look out on board for members of the Kyle Wide Club (Scotland's answer to the Mile High Club), whose ultimate challenge is the trip to Gigha.

An elderly nudist from Troon
Stayed out in the sun and got broon;
As he basked in the heather,
His skin changed to leather
And his cockle turned into a prune.

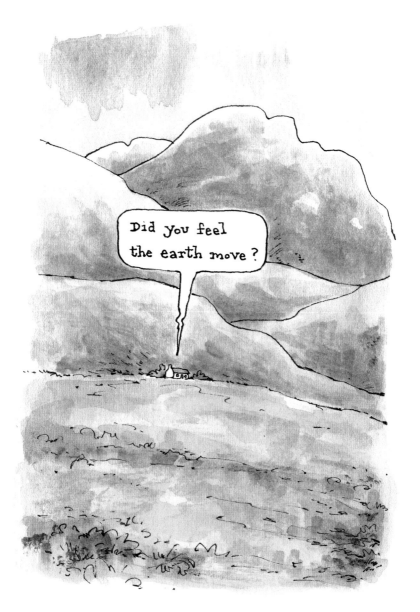

WESTERN ISLES

DRIVERS SHOULD REMEMBER to position their cars in the correct lanes for ferry embarkation to the Western Isles, with men on one side and women the other.

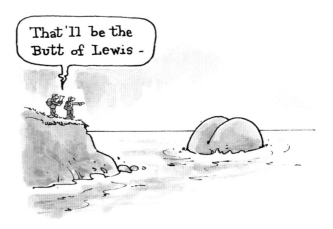

Scottish islands retain an air of ordered calm, far from the kind of troubles that beset their Greek and Spanish counterparts. All that could now change with global warming. Muckle Roe, Uist and Foula are some way still from Mykonos, Ibiza and Kos. Falkirk is not yet Faliraki. However, there are growing concerns for what may be to come in the way of all-night partying, collective sex and projectile vomiting in Highland resorts. Already the Scottish Tourist Board has taken the first steps in tightening checks on large parties heading north and in vetting their reps. Wallace Arnold, be warned.

A couple who lived near The Minch
Got stuck in a bedtime clinch;
To lever them free
Took ropes and a tree
Plus the loan of a nautical winch.

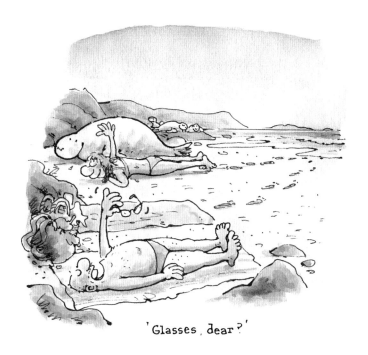

'Glasses, dear?'

NORTHERN ISLES

FOR THOSE who don't live there, Shetland and Orkney are easy to confuse. Both are off the map. One has sixty-seven islands (depending on the tide), the other claims more than a hundred; one has Papa Stour and Papa Little and the other has Papa Westray, Papa Stronsay, Papa Moomin and Sniff. In both the biggest island is Mainland, and both have a place called Twatt (also usually off the map). Both excel at place-names. Orkney has Hurliness and Grimness, Holms of Ire, Holm of Huip, Blotchnie and Spo, not to mention Holland and Ireland or Dishes and Work. Shetland has Mavis Grind and Flubersgerdie (distant cousins of Scapa Flo) and Noup of Noss and the Loch of Spiggie, along with traditional ailments Fitful Head and The Drongs, Grutness, Gloup and The Slithers.

Norse traditions still flourish in the Northern Isles, with Vikings Up-Helly-Aa-ing in the streets of Lerwick (wear wellingtons) and making the most of Shopping Week in Stromness. On Orkney is Skara Brae, the 4,500-year-old settlement (stone dresser, stone table, stone bed . . .) which has been the inspiration for many an off-piste B&B.

The Shetland Islands have a romantic past. Frau Stack, off Papa Stour, is a lonely rock on which a Viking lord is said to have put his only daughter, away from men, after she refused the marriage he had arranged. She survived her ordeal, somehow becoming pregnant in the course of it. Mousa Broch was where Thora Jewel-Hand honeymooned in the ninth century with Norwegian hubby Bjorn, driving everyone knuts with their dreadful music. Three centuries on, the same Mousa Broch was where Margaret of Atholl dallied with her Shetland toyboy, Erlend Ungi, while son Earl Harald laid siege outside. These days it would all get sorted on daytime TV.

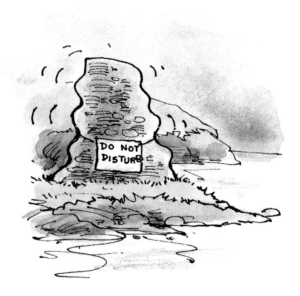

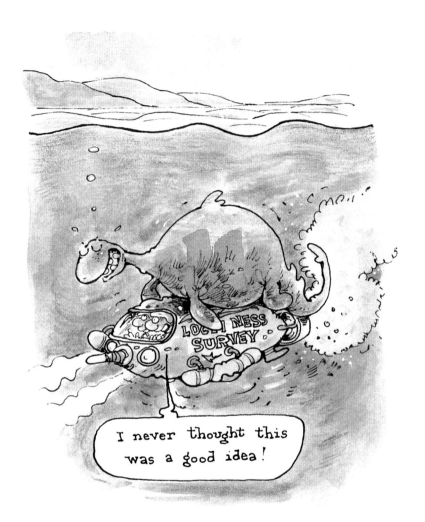

NORTH AND EAST

FAR FROM THE dour, grey place it is often made out to be, Scotland's north is a region buzzing with things of interest. Portmahomack, at the mouth of Dornoch Firth, has a fountain put up in 1887 to honour the arrival of Gravitational Water in the village. Along the Moray coast ('the Scottish Riviera') are the sands of Findhorn ('the Scottish Sahara'); beyond is Lossiemouth, birthplace of Ramsay MacDonald ('the Scottish Casanova') and Bangkok of the North. Up the road near Thurso is the northernmost branch of the Playboy Club, where the bunnies turn white in winter.

With the enthusiasm for which they are famous, Aberdonians have turned the Granite City into a place of pilgrimage for fun-lovers everywhere. The boom-town atmosphere owes much to the discovery and extraction of riches in the North Sea, where rigs are constantly at work, drilling for Scotch. The area behind Aberdeen is the last part of Scotland where Doric is spoken (a dialect of classical Greek and hangover from Enlightenment times, when Edinburgh was Athens of the North).

There's a spot on the coast called Footdee
At the edge of Aberdeen Cootdee.
'We love the sea air,'
Say residents there,
'Except when the weather is shootdee.'

SWIMWEAR
IN SCOTLAND

From the wide expanses of Sutherland (kindly emptied by the 1st Duke) down to the Border by Berwick, the east coast of Scotland is full of surprises. North Berwick was the scene of unusual goings-on in 1590, when two hundred witches (if such there be) were caught in the kirkyard at midnight, baring their breasts and queuing up to kiss the backside of their horned and hooved president – who was the Earl of Bothwell. That much, at least, was admitted by one of the participants – at the point of torture when her scalp was about to be parted from her skull. As the unfortunate Agnes Sampson and her story unravelled, details emerged of the role played by local schoolmaster John Fian. According to Newes from Scotland of 1591, Fian was a notable sorcerer and damnable doctor. He had earlier tried to seduce a local woman, engaging the young brother who shared her bed to 'obtaine for him three hairs of his sister's privities'. The boy failed in his task, handing over instead three hairs plucked from the udder of a young cow – which then vied for the sorcerer's affections.

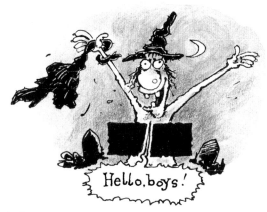

The whole matter was investigated personally by James VI, who held local witches to blame for his near shipwreck off the Bass Rock the previous May. He had seen them himself, transformed into hares and navigating a sieve, which circled his ship to whip up the storm. Burnings followed in Berwick. Up the coast at Dornoch, a stone marks the spot where Janet Horn was burnt at the stake in the 1720s, the last witch so to die in Scotland. She was accused of having turned her daughter into a pony and taken her to the Devil to be shod. Had she gone to the blacksmith, all might have been well.

A certain young lady in Berwick
Shared her bed with a neighbour called Derek,
Another called Peter,
Two men for the meter
And an elderly cleric named Eric.

The East Neuk of Fife has a special place in the dark annals. Dreel Castle was home in the eighteenth century to the Anstruther Dining Club, 'a Scottish Society of an erotic and convivial nature composed of the Nobility and Gentry of Anstruther'. It was more than a meeting-place for men who knew how to handle themselves; it was a mutual masturbation society (long before Channel Four). Don't ask about the jug passed round at the end of the meal. No mere flash in the pan, this society grew and grew. Members came together for more than a century and The Beggar's Benison, as it was known, went on to have branches in Glasgow, Edinburgh and St Petersburg. Dreel Castle is now a ruin.

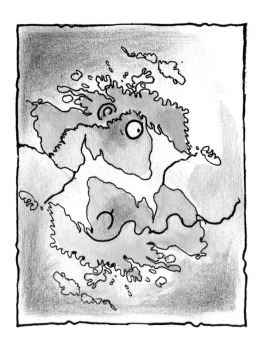

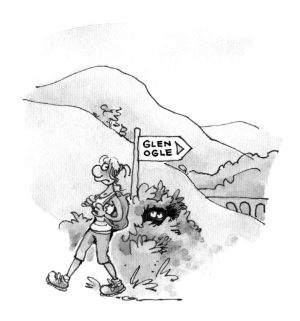

POPULAR HONEYMOON HIDEAWAYS

Ardaily, Auchtertool, Balkissock, Bonkle, Glenfeochan, Inverkip, Knockville, Moar, Isle of Ewe . . .

. . . and for the hardy: Stacks of Skroo (off the north coast of Fair Isle).

PLACE-NAMES IN NEED OF A RE-THINK

Bogend, Bogfields, Boghole, Dunbog, Dull, Dykehead, Gass, Grimness, Heck, Nitshill, Spittal, Stuck.

MORE SCOTTISH PLACE-NAMES IN NEED OF A RE-THINK

Pittendreich, Phorp, Spittal of Glenmuick, Yonder Bognie, Knabbygates, Strathbogie, South Cowbog, Duible, Cunside, Meikle Wartle, Bogfold, Flobbets, Backside and Whifflet.

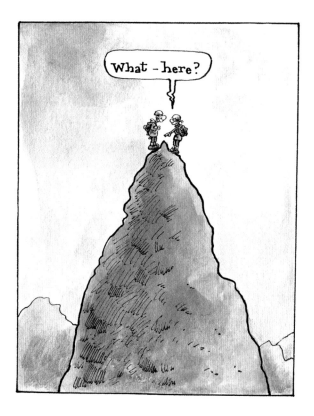

SCOTLAND'S SEXIEST MOUNTAIN

NOW THERE'S a topic for hot debate – and no shortage of stunners to line up for the title. A few stand out from the crowd, head and shoulders above the rest: Slioch, Suilven ('Scotland's Matterhorn') and shapely Stac Pollaidh. And then there are the regular knee-tremblers like Sgurr nan Gillean, moody An Teallach or graceful Ben Lui, dubbed 'Queen of Scottish Mountains'. Team entries are strong, as with the Three Sisters of Glencoe, not to be outdone by the Five Sisters of Kintail or the Paps of Jura. (Names do much for a mountain: one peak in the Cairngorms is Bod an Deamhain, which translates from the Gaelic as Devil's Penis, but is marked on maps as Devil's Point.)

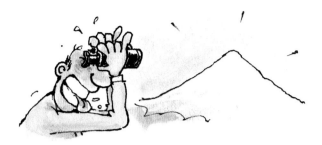

Maybe the crown should go to a surprise winner: step forward . . . Schiehallion (sob, gasp, flick back tears). Bang in the centre of Scotland, Schiehallion is modestly sized but perfectly formed. Such, at least, was the verdict of Charles Mason (he of the Mason-Dixon Line) in 1772. Mason had been sent north by the Royal Society to find the mountain in Britain with the most regular geometric shape, measurement of which would enable the Astronomer Royal to work out the weight (all right, mass) of the Earth. Two years later, Neville Maskelyne spent a wet and windy seventeen weeks on top of Schiehallion, directing teams of surveyors. The sums worked and Maskelyne got his answer. Best of all, one of the team found that by joining up figures that matched he had invented contours. And that is sexy, for a mathematician.

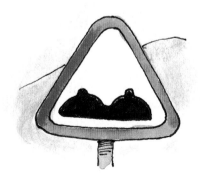

MODESTY PRESERVERS:

a selection of items obtainable by mail order from the Keep Scotland Decent Society

[specify tartan]

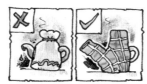

SAY GOODBYE TO TEATIME EMBARRASSMENT WITH THE NON-SUGGESTIVE

TEAPOT TROUSER

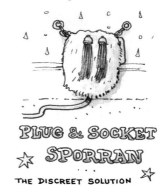

PLUG & SOCKET SPORRAN

☆ THE DISCREET SOLUTION ☆

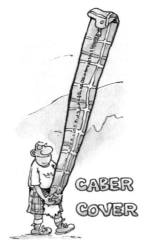

CABER COVER

NOZZLE SCREEN

available on request at Highland Filling-Stations

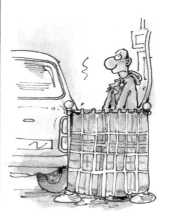

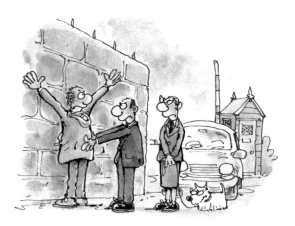

BORDER GUARDS ON THE LOOK OUT
FOR ILLEGAL IMPORT OF LEWD AND
LIBIDINOUS MATERIAL INTO SCOTLAND

4. For the Visitor

VISITOR ACCOMMODATION IN Scotland can be pretty particular. Bed and Breakfast means just that and nothing else, mind. Bedrooms are subject to regular inspection. It is not unusual to find beds fitted with car alarms as a deterrent to unseemly behaviour. Guests are expected to respect house rules and not to tarnish the reputation of the country. (For those arriving by air, the obligatory frisking at Prestwick may be the last such excitement for the duration of their stay in Scotland.) Anyone with half a mind bent on other things is encouraged instead to come by caravan. A menace on the roads, the mobile love-nest is nonetheless a blessing to all landladies who retain a proper sense of decency. Caravanners with unrestrained urges often make for the coast, where their private quarters may be seen, held down, for anti-rocking purposes, with stout ropes and large boulders. Among such visitors, the most sexually active are newly retired couples in campervans, who slink into lay-bys last thing at night. Always recognisable with their white beards, beige shorts and shiny thermos flasks, such folk are vital contributors to the economy of Scotland, not least in their consumption of tissues, marigolds and leisure goods.

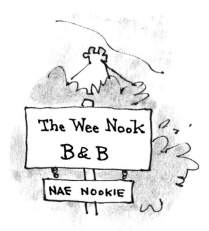

BED & BREAKFAST: THE EVENING RITUAL

NINE P.M. AND in the comfortable lounge (affording sea glimpses) of Mrs McCrumpet's Doss' n' Porridge Hoose, the clocks begin to chime. As the last strains of Korean electronic 'Scotland the Brave' sink into dralon cover and deep-pile carpet, a new sound is heard – the boinging of gong in the hall. Keys rattle in locks above and feet creak down the stairs, summoned – as bidden on first arrival – to the social event of the day: evening drinks at Mrs McCrumpet's.

First through the door is Finbar Sproat, sales representative, Scottish region. Sproat nabs the corner-seat, well hidden by rubber-plant, and settles back to study the field. Enter:

- a middle-aged man with darting eyes, on the run from unidentified penal institution
- two Americans, just happy to be here in Ireland
- a small family from Kent, smelling of car-sick and ready to kill
- one Serb, suited
- two lady cyclists from Holland, who have in the last twelve hours been over six Munros and taken in the view from Beinn Eighe, and are, even now, in rapid-fire Dutch, planning routes for the morrow
- one wobbly trolley, clinking with cups and laden with pots dressed as knitted Highlanders
- Mrs McCrumpet, with broad smile and tea-strainer.

'Has anyone seen the forecast?' starts Mrs McC.

'More rain sorry you–' three voices chime back in unison.

In the silence that follows, all eyes are drawn towards a small moth hurling itself against the velveteen drapes of a lampshade.

'Did somebody open their wallet?' beams Mrs McC.

The joke is repeated in all parts of the room, except around Sproat, who finds himself the object of piercing glares from two Dutch muscle-women. Choosing simple words and fluttering gestures, Sproat begins to explain the joke, but is cut short with a lecture in flawless English on the evils of national stereotyping.

With a long sigh, Sproat reaches for his cup of milky coffee, with wrinkling skin shortly due to transfer itself to his moustache. Into his pocket-book he pencils another nought and hopes, maybe, for a small change of fortune. Preferably in the next twenty-four hours, before he checks in to Sea Whispers, nr Oban, prop. N. McPhuttock (Mrs).

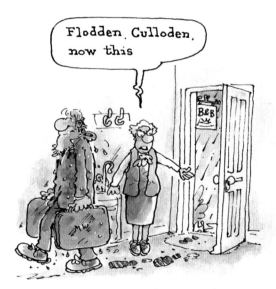

LEGENDARY HOSPITALITY

OFFICIAL WARNING SIGNS:

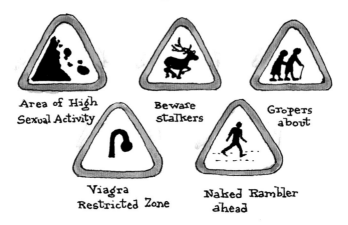

Area of High
Sexual Activity

Beware
stalkers

Gropers
about

Viagra
Restricted Zone

Naked Rambler
ahead

FOR FOREIGNERS

Correct approaches: how to say –

May I have a room for the night?
Have you space in your bed tonight?

May I inspect the bedroom?
Komm with me on the bed.

Thank you for your hospitality.
Please be grateful for our hostility.

I'm afraid the bedside lamp is not working.
My appliance does not function in your bed.

How nice – a ceilidh!
What's that frigging racket down below?

May I have the pleasure of the next dance?
Will you be 'aving the sex next with me?

We are unable to flush your loo.
You have big dung problems.

My husband is undergoing therapy for fetishism.
My husband will not come out of your drying-room.

Was that not a bidet?
We've not dared go near your wonderful display of local porcelain.

What a friendly dog – collie, is he?
Verflixter Scheisshund

Can I have an alarm call in the morning?
Please will you come frightening me in the bed tomorrow?

At eight o' clock.
You will be knocking me off for eight hundred hours.

US section:

What is the correct name in Scotland for a john?
John in Scotland is jock.

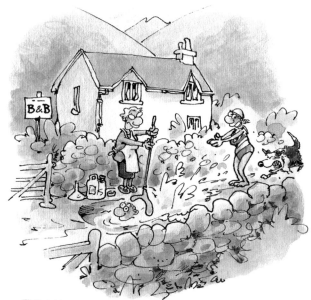

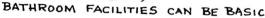

BATHROOM FACILITIES CAN BE BASIC

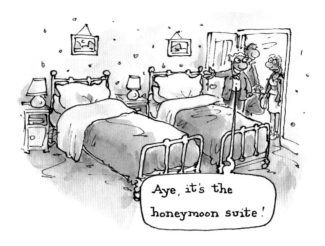

PREMARITAL RELATIONS

ONE EFFECTIVE WAY to preserve decency in the absence of spare bedrooms is the custom of 'bundling', traditional in Orkney and the Highlands as well as in the backwoods of colonial America. By this arrangement, a young man out courting was allowed to share the bed of his beloved, as long as she was 'bundled', i.e. sewn into a full set of clothes or trussed up in a bundling-bag and examined next morning. A further precaution could be had by the addition of a centreboard down the bed (spikes/ razor-wire optional). Unmarried couples visiting Scotland should check ahead whether their accommodation is in premises where bundling is still practised.

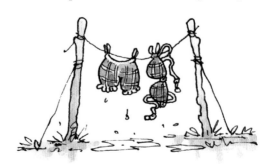

LINGERIE IN SCOTLAND

SCOTTISH CUSTOMS

Hogmanay, Whuppity Scourie, Rumpling the Haggis, Beltane, Beef Brose and Shriften E'en, Hunt the Gowk, Cold-sore Monday, Up Helly-Aa, Withersgreip, Gropefast, Ramgiblet, Stotefimble, Preen-tail Day, Ba Game, Sowans Nicht . . .

Scotland has a rich tradition of seasonal festivities, customs and special occasions. Most involve darkness, fumblings and a wonderful hangover next day. Chief of these is Hogmanay, celebrated over several nights in city streets, with pavement performances.

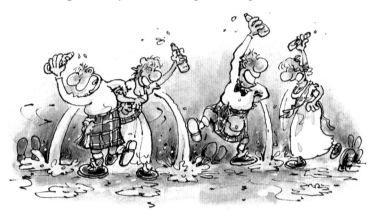

MEMBERS OF THE REAL WHITE HEATHER CLUB SEE IN THE NEW YEAR

Different places find different ways of celebrating. Burghead sees the Burning of the Clavie; in Stonehaven they set fire to their balls. On Lewis it is necessary for a boy dressed in a sheepskin to walk clockwise round the fire (increasingly difficult in modern houses). Elsewhere survive similar rituals, such as dressing up in cattlehides and running round the village being beaten by sticks. There are many forms of enjoyment.

Common to all is the good-luck rite of First Footing. The first to cross the threshold, once the clock has struck midnight, must be a tall, dark, handsome (optional) stranger, bearing gifts of whisky, shortbread, bannocks, salt and a piece of coal – Scots will eat anything by this stage of the evening. Few manage all ingredients; most make do with a fast emptying scottle of botch and a handful of something moist and brown.

Blond Viking types, hell-bent on pillage and rape, are not welcomed through the door at such times; by tradition, they spend the evening in, with a packet of crispbread and plateful of fish parts.

The name Hogmanay is said to come from the Early Flemish 'Hoouargghh-mnn-aieecchh', the sound of neighbours throwing up in the road outside.

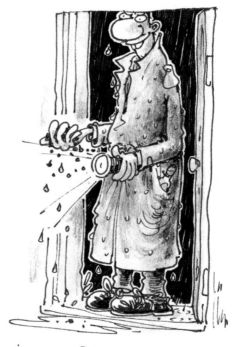

... something moist and brown.

Dates for your Diary:

1 Jan   Dufftown Boys' Walk (rest of Scotland ill in bed)
25 Jan   Haggis Mating Season starts
18 Oct   Sour Cakes Day
31 Oct   Nut Crack Night

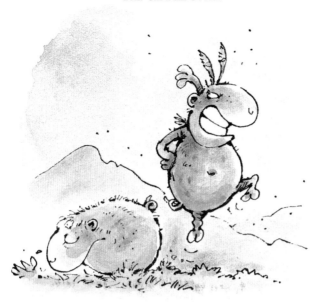

COURTING RITUAL OF THE HAGGIS

COURTING TRADITIONS

To find out more about your future partner:

Slice the peel off an apple, all in one go. Wait till midnight, then whirl it round your head. As the clock strikes twelve, chuck the peel over your left shoulder. The shape it lands in will form the first letter of the name of the one you will marry. It will be someone whose name begins with S.

Up in Orkney:

Every part of the world has its own marriage customs – Mexican newlyweds each have a rope put around the neck. But few can compete with Orkney when it comes to wedding ritual, from Speirin to Hame Fare, Blackening to Back Feast, Kissing Meat to Kirking. The marriage should take place at a time of waxing moon, on a Thursday, but not in

May or when the football is on. After Fit Washing Night the used water (or Blue Nun, if posh) should stand out in sunlight for twelve hours, but not be looked at by a dog. The 'cog' drunk by the bride consists of:

> 2 bottles of whisky
> 2 bottles of rum
> 1 bottle of brandy
> 1 bottle of gin
> 1 bottle of port
> 3 pints of stout
> 12 pints of home-brew
> warmed with sugar and mixed spices

A similar thing is done on Fridays in Glasgow, without the sugar and

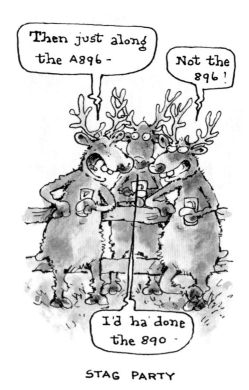

STAG PARTY

EASILY CONFUSED :

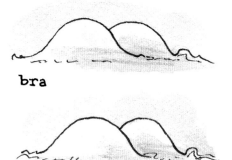

bra

brae

spices.

One of those and an Orkney bride is up for anything.

SCOTTISH WORDS THAT DON'T MEAN WHAT YOU THINK THEY MIGHT

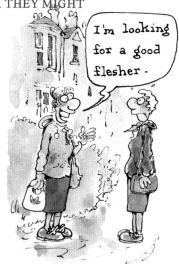

I'm looking for a good flesher -

awee	a moment
biggin	building
birk	birch tree
dyke	low stone wall
feck	amount, majority
flesher	butcher
forfochen	exhausted
goolie	knife
grape	grope
guid-willy	generous
haugh	water meadow
poke	paper bag
shak	shake
tittie	little sister
vyce	voice
willie-goo	herring-gull or lout

THOSE POSTCARDS:

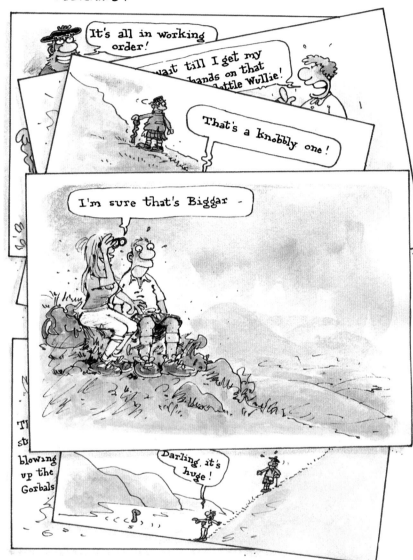

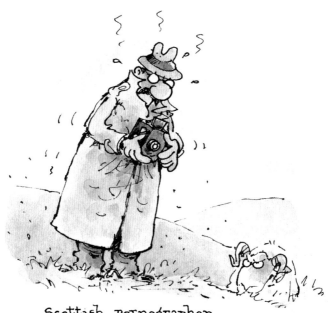

Scottish pornographer
out in the field

5. Scotland's Porn Industry

ONCE A THRIVING CONCERN, the Scottish porn industry is now in sad decline. From small beginnings, with weekly collections by travelling salesmen from isolated crofts in the Highlands and Islands, the business saw massive growth in the course of the nineteenth century. By the end of Victoria's reign, whole communities were engaged in its production and achieving global distribution. From the east coast ports large fleets sailed out each season, laden with creels for southern markets. The railways, too, did their bit for Scottish output, fast-tracking fresh porn deliveries to the breakfast tables of the capital.

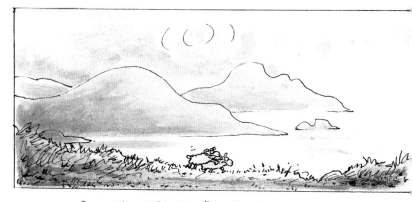

from The Colin Baxter Hardcore Range

It was the spread of the Internet in the 1990s which did for the industry and output reduced to a trickle. There is little home-grown porn to be found out on top shelves these days – most is shipped straight off to Spain. However, it often pays to ask discreetly, under the counter.

BLUE MOVIES OF SCOTLAND: (28) CERTIFICATE

Hot in Hawick
Confessions of a Sheep Dipper
Last Tango in Harris
Deep Groat
The Ups and Downs of a Bandy Ram
120 Days of Selkirk
Crieff Encounter
Belle de Jura
Callander Girls
A Man and a Wumman

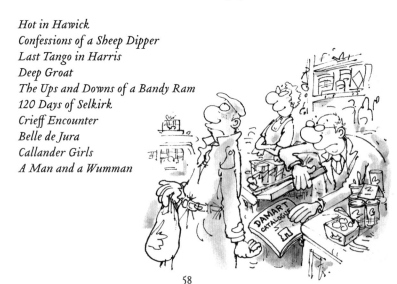

SHOPPING

S COTLAND IS WELL supplied with sex shops. These are called 'Camping' or 'Outdoor Equipment' stores, and purvey rubberwear, leather goods and accessories to excite all tastes. As a rule, the further north you go, the wilder the appetite of customers you may encounter and the more specialised the goods. Fort William has long been recognised as a world centre for bondage equipment. Do not be afraid to ask assistance for items you seek that are not on display.

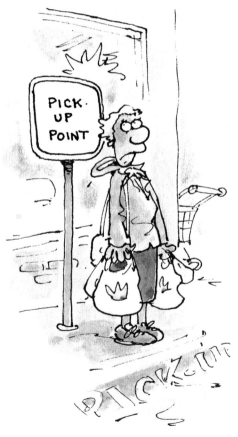

LIVE ENTERTAINMENT

L ARGS, CRINAN, MALLAIG, Uig, Plockton, Scourie, Peterhead, Pittenweem . . . Scotland's ports cannot compete in size with the likes of Amsterdam or Hamburg, but they more than make up for this in charm and individuality. Red-light districts tend to be marked out more discreetly than around the world and strict rules of Sunday Observance prevail in many parts, more especially the west. Check ahead for opening hours of Swingers' Clubs around Stornoway.

There is no great tradition of striptease in Scotland (or 'peel-aff', as it is on neon signs), but this is largely down to the weather. Lap-dancing ('sporran-care') flourishes mainly in clubs and establishments for private members only. For pole-dancing, jigs and reels, look out for premises hosting traditional Scottish dance events. Always check for legality. In 1874 a Free Church minister from Argyll prosecuted one of his elders for participating in a Scottish reel at a ball.

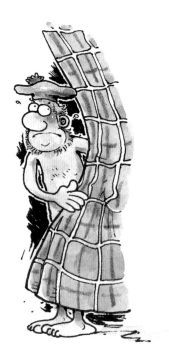

6. The Joy of Sets

Lesson one: Getting started
As experienced couples know, there are many different ways of having fun on the floor. Before attempting to strike lucky with a Gay Gordon or learning how to Roger de Coverley, absolute beginners should familiarise themselves with a few basic moves: set-to, face up, cast-off, drop, cross over, change places, swing together, reel, retire . . .

Lesson two: Positions
Practise simple positions: dosi-do, elbow grip, petronella, groin clutch, tongue lock, poussette . . .

Homework: The Seann Triubhas (pronounced 'shawn trews'): trad dance depicting a Scotsman shedding his trousers.

Lesson three: A simple jig
Now you are ready to try a Ladies' Fancy.
Do this first at home, in the company of
a few close friends:

- First man turns second woman
  with right hand and returns
  to position
- First couple turn by left
  hand and finish with two
  hands, first man giving
  left hand to second woman
  and right hand to partner
- Lead down the middle and
  back up to places
- First two couples give
  four hands across then back
- Both pairs poussette
  and repeat

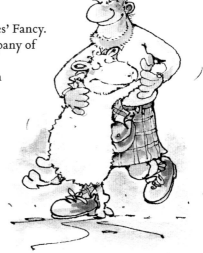

Enjoy that? Now for something a little more adventurous.

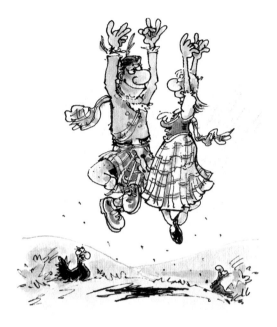

Lesson four: 'The Dog's Deid' (Strathspey)
Suitable tunes: 'Awa' on the Brae', 'The Milkman's Cumming', 'McHaddock's Lament' . . .

- Couples face up and set to
- First lady bounces on supporting foot, pointing with leading leg
- First man leads off, stepping on to first lady's foot
- Lady turns on him, man retires
- Second couple swing together, arch, turn, sideslip to bottom
- Third couple clench buttocks and allemande
- Fourth couple basket and peak
- First couple cross hands, change places and look around for help
- Second couple cast off and purl
- Third and fourth couples triangle en croute, then cast off to bottom
- First couple repeat swing, man leads left, right, left, kick
- Lady spins, bloody furious
- Men retreat behind the furniture

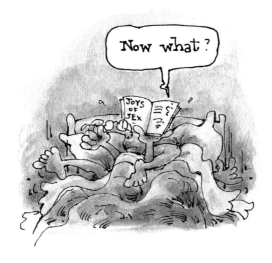

TECHNIQUES

Hard to Get
Female sends Christmas card, then chains door, closes shutters and bars every entrance. Takes phone off hook, switches off mobile and retires to bath. Continues indefinitely.

Cock o' the North
Large testosterone-fuelled male circles female in open space, strutting his stuff with head held high, chest puffed out and full display of manpower; voice varied, with dark mutterings and high-pitched whistles interspersed with noises like popping corks and drum-rolls. Female responds with disparagement, scornful brays and cackles. Continues thus a good while. Finally roused to uncontrolled frenzy, male leaps on female from behind. Seconds later, is gone for good. Method used by capercaillie.

Loch Fyne
Only when there is an R in the month.

Sheepdog

Handler stands at post with whistle in hand to issue basic commands: left go-by, right-away to me, stop, walk straight-up and come-by. Partner does best to oblige.

Speyside

Lengthy and protracted ritual in classic stages (dressing, grinding, worm-tub, still, nosing, tasting) that can take up to twelve years to complete.

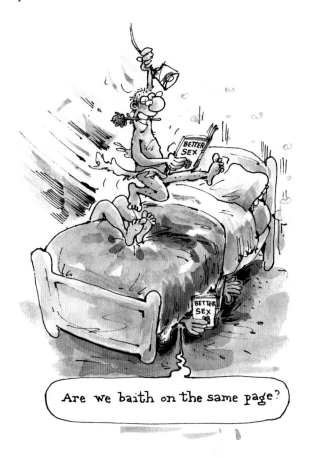

Are we baith on the same page?

The Rut

Before the dark evenings set in, males appear in excitable state, parading their assets and displaying their wares. Around them gather circles of admiring females. The one that trumpets most, has the biggest biceps, flashiest Mondeo and largest following, is deemed prize stud and winner takes all. Losing males slink off dejected.

North Sea Crude

Hard drilling in the dark accompanied by much effing and blinding.

West Highland Way

Gruelling procedure requiring protective outer wear (hoods, waterproof trousers, etc.) regular breaks and a high level of fitness.

Vertical Ascent

Approach, traverse, glissade, exposure, zipper effect, Cheyne-Stokes phenomenon, depth hoar, self-arrest, French technique . . . the world of mountaineering has a rich terminology to cover every position or eventuality, from first ascent to final assault. Beginners should not try these moves except under guidance and well roped together. Essential equipment: harness, dark glasses, Kendal mint-cake, oxygen.

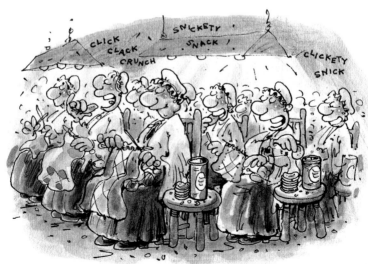

BEHIND THE SCENES AT PRINGLE SWEATERS

SEX AIDS

Kilt hose; fly plaid; pacamac; sporran strap; spurtle; tartan flashes; midge hood; Millar's Pan Drops; traffic cone; see-through cagoule; knobkerrie; niblick; diamond-pattern golfing sweater; Walnut Whip; Caramel Log.

NB: Protectives in Scotland ('wee bunnets') follow traditional patterns of styling, finished off with diced band and feather or pom-pom, as required. When buying at a chemist's, it is usual to state preference (balmoral, glengarry or tam) along with clan affiliation.

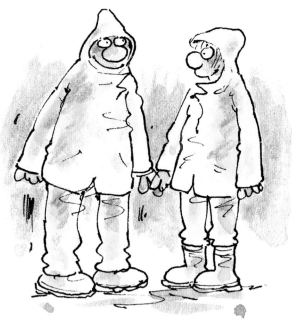

safe sex

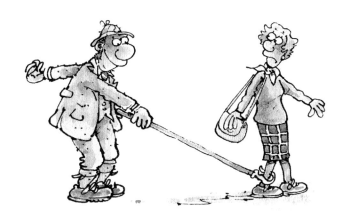

Finding the Perfect Partner

LONELY HEARTS COLUMN: TERMINOLOGY EXPLAINED

term	means	but could mean
gsoh	genuine Scot on heat	gosh, I'm dyslexic
wltm	would like to mate	with little to mention
ltr	long-term rumpy-pumpy	long-term regret
sim int	simple interest	simian intellect
n/s	non sniffer	nits sufferer
outdoor type	homeless	keeps ferrets
fun-loving	alcoholic	collects whoopee cushions
enjoys opera	pretentious	watches *Neighbours*
cultured/cultivated	can use knife and fork	druggie
enjoys walking	disqualified from driving	unable to run
likes dogs	up for rough sex	covered in dribble and doghairs

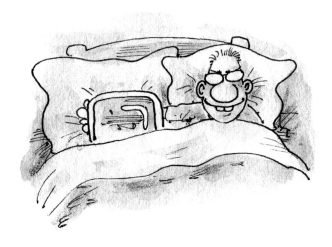

COMPUTER DATING

THE DEVELOPMENT of the microchip has revolutionised the world of distance dating. Gone are the days of love-lorn souls on distant islets or lonely hilltops, waving their flags in the mist. The system depended on mastery of semaphore, incomplete knowledge of which often gave rise to misunderstandings. All that has been superseded by the slick, fast world of cybersex.

That First Fond Email:

Dear Cutie of Cumbernauld,

Wot a wiked repply. You can come and fry my onoins any day. No size deosn't mater who cares more the merier as the bishpo said to the arctress. I too am verry fond of oprah, fine wines and good littracher so we shoulkd get on like a mouse on fire I loom forward to meating you.

Your shinning nit in amour, Wee J.

PS Are you m or f?

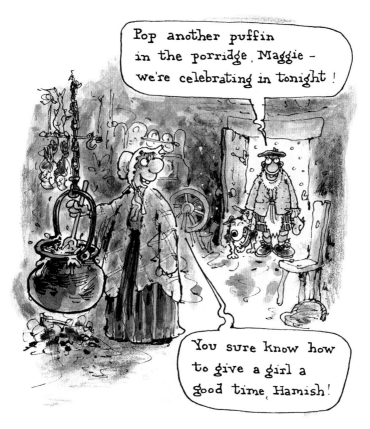

LIFE WAS HARD IN FORMER TIMES

From Early Manuals

For conceiving of a boye

Tak 3 pyne-needles togither wythe ye tongues of 24 moles, mixed with parslie, and ye spleen of 1 whelk, warmed in 2 gills of mylke from a red cow and place by quartyr moon in ye husband's usuall portion of ye maritle bedde. Do this privilye, switche on ye radio and waite.

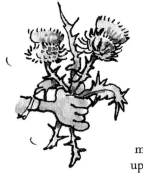

For prevencioune of pregnancie
Weave gurdle of ye finest threads of sylke, flakks, maidenhair fern and thongweed, cunnyngly constructing as ye go a concealedde chamber within for placement of ye head of one thistle. Goe about yore busynesse with all-daye confydence, exceptyng should ye, less mindful of yore inner secrette, mounte upon an orse.

For makkyng of bairns
Firstlie to improve ye seminal vigours, be sure to hytte the toone of a goodlie houre on a Fryday nicht therebye best to get well bladdyrd on 10 pyntes of Red Bull, Lagerr Toppe, McEwenne's etc followd by ye usual shortts and thenne ye payvement outpourrings in reddinesse for ye bisnesse.

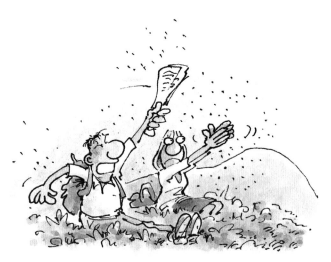

slap and tickle in the heather

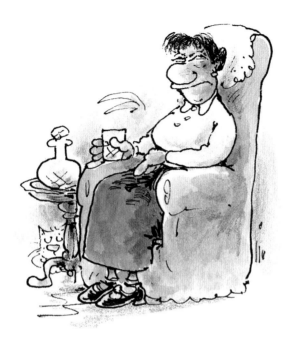

The Listening Ear

PRACTICAL ADVICE FROM NOREEN MCNARGLE,
THE SCOTTISH NANNY WITH THE NO-NONSENSE ANSWERS

Q. I seem to be having difficulties with the ole waterworks at present, giving problems with bedtime and you-know-what. Can you help?

One quart of water in regular sips before each meal, followed by good plain food, properly boiled. You will find plenty of ideas in my best-selling book of nursery treats, 'No Nice Pudding Till You've Finished That First' (pub. Friggett & Bawles of Bloomsbury).

Q. My hubby of seven years has become hopeless at cuddles. He hasn't forgotten how to, as I've seen him do it with others (e.g. Maureen in Sales). What can I do?

Och, you puir milksop. Was it mollycoddles that made the British Empire? I think not. What you want in a man is firm strength and well-creased underpants. Now away with your nonsense.

Q. I am 61 and very ignorant about sex – how can I find out more?

Me too. We should get together.

Q. My partner and I are deeply in love and see eye-to-eye on all things, except at meals, when he makes loud sucking noises over the soup. It is threatening our marriage – what can be done?

In my day you would haul him out by the ear and bang his head hard against the bannister until the little toerag was ready to learn some manners. You aren't supposed to do that these days, so I would make sure the front door is locked first.

Q. I followed your advice last month with regard to the figs and the tubing, but am not sure which way up the tarpaulin should go.

Mr McSlipper & Friends for you.

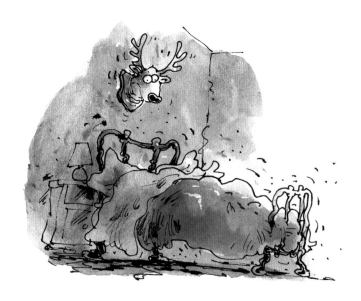

Sex Education in Scotland

YOU'LL NO' BE NEEDING ANY OF THAT!

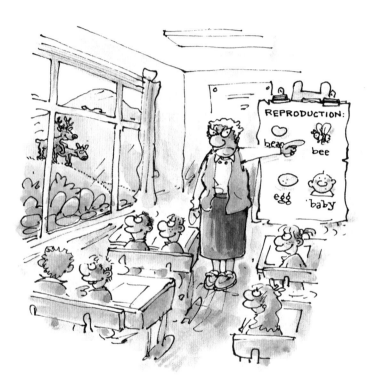

NOWHERE IN BRITAIN has Sex Education ever played a large part in the school curriculum. Sex was placed firmly in the category of things best left unsaid. At least one girls' school in the 1950s roped off its pond early each year to protect the pupils from the sight of frogs mating. Children in city primary schools, deprived of the sights of the countryside, might be led to the park on a Nature Walk, returning with a paper bag containing something nasty for the Nature Table.

It was up in the secondary schools that biology lessons really took off. Children were given broad beans to cut open and expected to work things out from there. Then, in the 1970s, along came That Film, the one with teachers in bed, doing things undreamt of by Miss Jean Brodie (or maybe not). The very thought of teachers (or, worse, their own teachers) engaging in such practices was so foul that many young folk were successfully put off sex for life. Back to the broad bean it was.

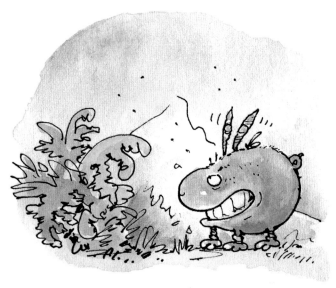

HAGGIS ON THE PULL

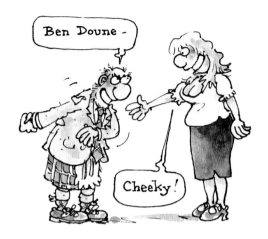

Chat-Up Lines in Scotland

- Can I tempt you to a shortbread finger?
- That's a fine-looking thing in your sporran
- Lovat?
- Can I buy you half a drink?
- Ye'll no' ravish me, the noo
- Your tartan?
- Will ye no' share a posset wi' me?
- Are you up for the stalking?
- Is this the right way to Ogil?
- Ben Doune!
- Come up and see my itchings (midge season only)
- Is that something you've got in the Trossachs?
- There's more rain forecast
- How can I get to Poolewe?
- I've no' had the pleasure
- Join me in a Highland Fling?
- Have I not seen you on Grampian?
- D'ye have the time?
- Have you not seen my Eightsome Reel?
- They do an awfu' good ceilidh here later
- (Festival time) When are you on?

75

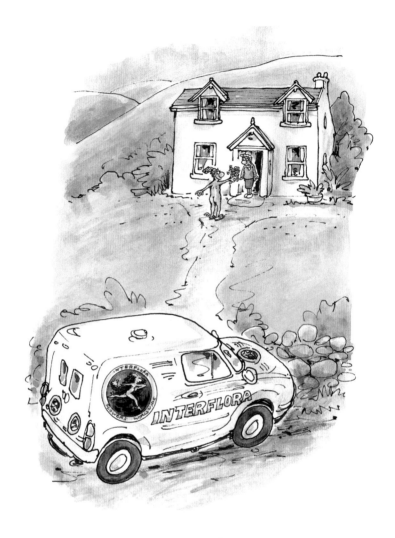

Foreplay

- That you, Maggie?

- It's a braw nicht –

Terminology

Act of Union
aka Highland Fling, getting familiar, something untoward, southern ways, Festival behaviour, none of that here, houghmagandy, annual service, warming yourself up, peltin, excuse me, no-score draw, the Auld Alliance, Scots Wha' Hae', mowe, winching

Oor Wullie
aka Wee Jimmy, The Old Firm, the Member for Fife, cockle, winkle, the Old Man of Hoy, the Inaccessible Pinnacle, dokey, the Trossachs, boaby, bubbly-jock, the Gorbals, Mick McManus, Wee Willie Winkie, dibber, dobber, Mr McGregor, the 5th Duke of Gordon (Cock o' the North), Big Mac, the Monarch of the Glen, puir wee thing, tassle, tossle, tadger, todger, pintle, whang

Lassie
aka hen, hinnie, coo, tottie, chuckie, stoater, doxy, tart, shelter belter, wifie, wumman, wee besom, quean

Ladies' Excuse Me
aka Fingal's Cave, Kyle of Lochalsh, Queen o' the South

Words Used by English Folk Pretending to be Scots
ach, och, ich, ech, uch, aye, lief, numpty, bonny, outwith, bampot, teuchter, wee, sassenach

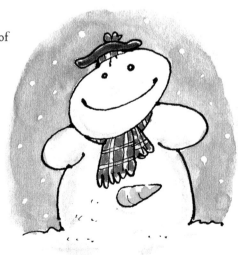

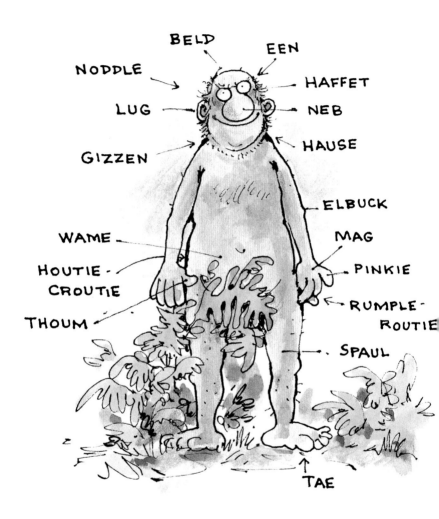

THE BODY BEAUTIFUL :
KNOW YOUR PARTS.

For That Special Evening

This recipe comes from Marcel of the Four Drainpipes, one of Scotland's leading fooderies.

Surprised Lamb a l'Ecossaise

Material for 2 persons:

1 coast of lamb (or can be done with mouse of lamb)
6 large turnups
heart and lungs of cabbage
1 branch of celery
1 oignon nailed with cloves
1 freshly raped carrot
2 pluches of thyme and 1 of parsley
6 cloves of garlic
40g alleged butter
8 cloves of garlic
953 ml water
1 bottle of Scotch

Service:

Lamb disgusts itself best before the arrival of spring. Sheep can be serviced in all manner of interesting fashion, from perfume with cumin to light watering with grateful cheese.

Method:

First harrass your lamb for several minutes before flash-burning on lively fire for 40 seconds. Do this en cocotte with finger of butter and then retire under blanket. Divide the branch of celery and hack into small districts. Fill a marmite and boil to bring. Add coast of lamb with prepared vegetables and powder with chiselled parsley. Go and sit in a warm oven for 5 hours. The lamb will cook itself, molesting gently from time to time. One hour before termination, excite the lamb with a wooden spoon. Add cabbage and garlic, with peppering from a new windmill. At last minute, give summer and winter to tasteful, and varnish with parsley. Add Scotch. Accompany with potatoes, baker's wife, butter and bowels of greenery. Enjoy à deux.

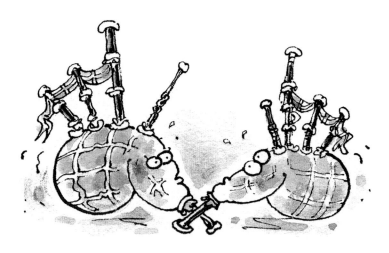

BAGPIPES MATING

7. Literature & Art

IN LITERATURE AND art, Scotland has its fair share of earthy subjects and steamy passages, though few have escaped the blue pencil of the censor. The earliest known examples go back to *The Minstrel Lays*.

TENDER MOMENTS IN SCOTTISH WRITING

A heron flapped up fra' the long pool beyond the birks. In the chill of the gloaming, McTavish's daughter lay back in the heather, watching thin spirals of steam curl up from the man's outstretched withers.

'Tha's gander bree auchter the stoots,' he grumbled.

And she sighed a long sigh, as deep as Loch Snoddy . . .

from the 1930s semi-classic, *Gwen o' the Glen* by Glaven Bantry

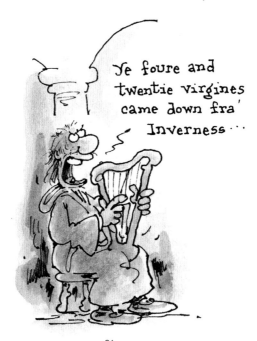

A rustle of silk in the darkness and he felt his tawse stiffen uncomfortably. Her hand lingered on his snib.

'Tha's gangin' awa?' she quivered.

'Glaikit,' he croaked.

And she mithered aneen. Soft fingers of moonlight caressed the white form of her gobbins. Outside, an otter called in the inky stillness.

'Braveness, ma wee hinnie,' he added, with sudden resolution, and a tremor ran down the plaid curtain she clung on to.

The Moon i' the Shutter by Barbara Gobes Cornforth
(runner-up in the Farquahar Prize for Romantic Friction, 1964)

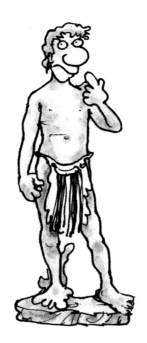

LOST MASTERPIECES
OF SCOTTISH ART:
McElangelo's 'David'

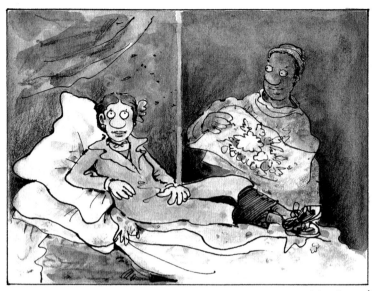

LOST MASTERPIECES OF SCOTTISH ART : McManet's Olympia

10 Aug 1887

Dire Dearie,

I've tracked a punk and billed two fags. Tomorrow we leave for
Sconny Botland. First we take the drain to Tumfries, kipping out of
Slumberland as our marriage cakes its way into Gretna. We plan to get
as far north as we can - Wart Filliam certainly, if not Muckle Flugga
(which may be just as well).

13 Aug
We have found charming lord and bodging in Miss McClootie's wee
abode ('Nosy Cook') just outside Bumdarton. Last evening found us
in Glasgow with much commotion in the streets following a game of
bootfall (Roath Ravers v Thartick Pistle). We took our pleasure instead
with an evening stroll beside the river, enjoying the ever-inviting but
womb-laden daughters of the Clyde.

14 Aug
We taught a pony and crap to the station and boarded a train for the north. Alas, our engine broke down as it entered a tunnel, but my neighbour entertained his fellow-passengers by pulling a cunning little stunt - no doubt his tarty prick. With great ingenuity, he had balanced a small potato on the end of his nose and the louder we all laughed, the more indignant the face he pulled. The fun lasted more than two hours. However, when he left the train at our next halt, I could not help noticing it was no potato, but a natural protuberance. Ho-heigh.

17 Aug
Today we passed Knock Less, but no sign of the Nonster Messy. Just time for a dick quip, then on to Inverness and a grand treat in the dining-room of McTavish's Hostelry. The gong sounded, dyed whores opened up and the gran of the hoose wheeled in a freshly shot mouse.

18 Aug
Attended kirk and made the acquaintance of Rev. McTatter, clan of the moth and vocal licker. We passed an enjoyable hour exchanging ales and tissues of mutual interest.

20 Aug
A lengthy moorland tramp on foggy ways to admire the balls of Glomach. Encountered en route a naturalist out bagging turds, some of which later, he confided, would be shot for his collection. On our return we accepted his invitation to bop dry and view his magnificent display, lovingly preserved in class gases. Varmellous.

Spoctor Dooner's Trottish Scavels:
From *Extracts from a Jittery Learn-all.*

'Whitthef--------------dy---b----f----!'
'C----the------f----g------f----?'
'----- me.'

Drainspitting by Mervyn Belch

Fo, Edinburgh it if, a place much given to Purfuit of Wantonneff and Pleafure. Notwithftanding itf Propenfity to the Vices and Follies of fafhionable Tranfgreffion, thif Town produces Ladies of erect Deportment and uncommon Beauty and it if our noble Tafk to preferve them from Attempts upon their Virtue. Our Men efpy an House of Infamy, wherein fome Ladies do their Bufinefs, and in a frame of Publick Spirit we enter in to remonftrate and succour. It if a Matter of fome Hours before we leave thif accurfed Spot, all infected with the Itch and Scab, the very Sight of which being sufficient to give a well-bred Dog the Vapours. And yet it bore Accreditation and Insignia of ye Scottish Tourift Board, three Stars to wit, compleat with Toafting-Fork and Troufer-Prefs.

A Compleat Account of the late Rebellion,
as It Occurr'd to Me by Ocular Demonftration
by A Volunteer, 1745

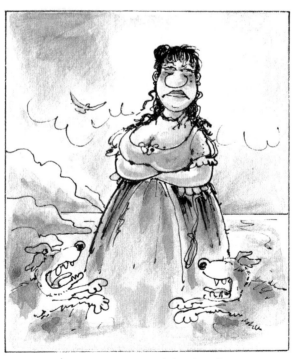

'SLAG AT BAY' by Landseer.

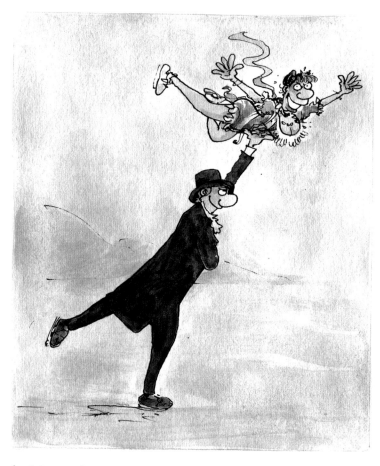

LOST MASTERPIECES -

Sir Henry Raeburn, early study for
Rev Robert Walker Skating on Duddingston Loch

SCOTLAND IN VERSE

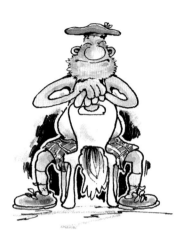

A beast by the name of McTavish
Led a life both sinful and lavish:
With gifts of large pearls
He trapped simple girls
Whom then he proceeded to ravish.

A roofer from near Ballachulish
Was made to look rather foolish
What he thought well-built
In the realm of his kilt,
The crowd below reckoned quite ghoulish.

An eminent gent from Tranent
Was generally thought a bit bent;
His favourite ruse
Was pleasuring ewes
In a secret inflatable tent.

A well-endowed barmaid from Leuchars
Had breasts sticking out like bazookas;
To admirers - and mockers
She explained that her knockers
Owed all to her fondness for Deuchars.

The beloved of one from Arbroath
Remarked as he plighted his troth,
That thing neath your kilt
Shows no hint of wilt
But signs of remarkable growth.

There was a young lady of Tain
Who fancied it now and again,
And again and again,
Again and again,
Again and again and again.

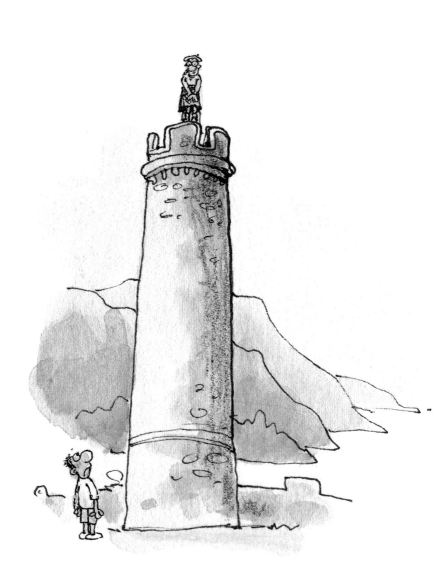

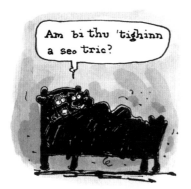

8. Get by in Gaelic

USEFUL PHRASES

Seall dè fhuair mi	Look what I've got
Co leis a tha seo?	Whose is this?
Leig às e	Let go of it
Gabhaidh mi am fear seo	I'll take this
Dè rinn thu?	What have you done?
Tha toll air	It's got a hole in it
Dè seòrsa rud a tha thu 'lorg?	What sort of thing are you looking for?
Tha mi dìreach a' coimhead	I'm just looking
Am bi thu 'tighinn a seo tric?	Do you come here often?
Mo chreach!	My goodness!
Dè tha thu 'dèanamh?	What are you doing?
Foghnaidh sin	That's enough
Chan eil e gu mòran feum	It's not much use
Chan eil e 'freagairt	It doesn't fit
Bha e cho mòr ri seo . . .	It was this big . . .
A bheil fear eile agaibh?	Have you got another one?
Feumaidh tu tionndadh a dhol an rathad eile	You'll need to turn and go the other way
Greas ort	Hurry up
Tha mi 'leigeil m'anail greiseag	I'm having a rest for a minute
Nach eil thu 'fàs sgìth dheth?	Aren't you getting tired of it?
Chòrd sin rium glan	I really enjoyed that
Obh obh!	Oh no!

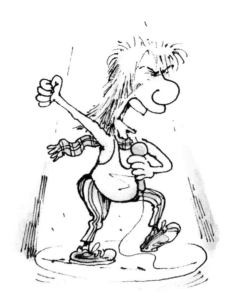

SEX·GODS OF SCOTLAND:
ROD STEWART (son of Andy)

9. The Music of Love

SEX UNLEASHED: THE STORY OF SCOTTISH POP

N O ACCOUNT OF popular music in Scotland would be complete
without mention of Archie Moncrieff, the Maestro of Mirth.
The young Archibald first came to prominence in the music-
halls of the 1870s with his unusual act featuring two turnips and a deft
hand on the *slibonneach* (trad Gaelic instrument closely related to the
Balinese nose-pipe). Moncrieff's act, unchanged over sixty years,
always began with him bounding on to the stage to pat his sporran and
call to the audience, 'Ye'll niver guess whit's under here –' As the
audience dried their tears, he would then whip out his unusual
instrument and proceed to perform a series of lively jigs and
traditional ballads, all to his own accompaniment. It was a routine

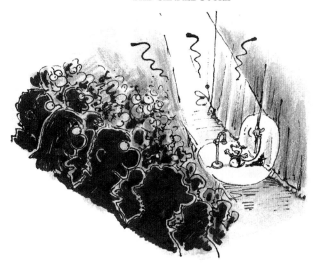

SHEP THE SINGING COLLIE

that won him huge acclaim, from workers' club to Windsor Castle. Success in Variety brought Sir Archibald more and more roles on the stage, most famous of all being that of Puir Wee Jimmie in Mrs Hartley Letwynde's evergreen tearjerker, *Crabbit Hoose*. This was the part that gave Moncrieff all those wonderful lines he made his own – many still in daily use. 'There's nae cake i' the tin, mither', 'There's nae kail in the yard, mither', 'There's nae peat o' the fire, mither' . . . delivered always with that doleful shake of the head. National catchphrases, these proved great morale boosters over two world wars. In retirement, Moncrieff, who hailed from Esher, returned to the family estates in Surrey, emerging regularly to be spotted in the Members' Enclosure at Epsom. His funeral in 1932 was an occasion of great mourning, notable for the cry that went up from the crowd as his coffin was drawn from the hearse: 'Ye'll niver guess whit's under here!'

The first half of the twentieth century was the heyday of the music hall in Scotland. Variety was king and bills shone with a galaxy of stars: Orlando and his Coloured Dove; Semprenata Sweet, the Lassie from Leith; Hamish McFee and his Halfpenny Whistle; Bing Broon, the Crooner from Troon; Kilbride Orpheans; Jock McStrap ('A Song, a Dance and a Sleight of Hand Mystification'); Nellie Wormald and

Patch; Ojnab Llib, the Man Who Sang Backwards; Don ('Highland Laundry Blues') Coatbridge, the Lad from Lanarkshire, on knee-fiddle and spoons; Raymondo and his All Stars; the Human Billiard Table; Bess of Barlinnie; Shep the Singing Collie . . .

The Twenties and Thirties saw in a bright new age of fun and frivolity. From Foulbog to Findhorn, Scottish flappers were out dancing each night, till 9.30 or later. Radio and the wind-up gramophone brought huge followings to the likes of Chico Airdrie and the Rhythm Boys; Mario Lochranza, the Scottish Tenor; and Googie Rothes and the Peterhead Palm Court Orchestra.

Then Rock shook the world. It was an unprecedented explosion of pent-up teenage energy, vigour, moodiness, sex and rage that erupted over the Fifties and Sixties. America had Little Richard, Jerry Lee Lewis and Elvis the King. England had Marty Wilde, Adam Faith, Billy Fury. And Scotland had Kenneth McKellar.

The Presleys left Scotland in 1745.

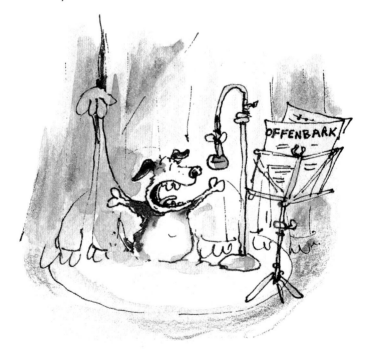

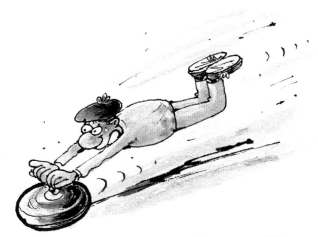

10. Sport for All

Essential Equipment
Gloves, stopwatch, bagpipes, addis mop, curling-pants, non-matching shoes (teflon-coated slider and latex rubber brake-shoe or tartan slipper and gumboot, court shoe and running spikes etc.), thermos, curling tongs.

Bewildering Terminology
Wick, hack, hammer, blank end, in-handle, hollow grind, out-handle, split guard.

History
Believed to date back many centuries to the time when men were men and winters cold. A local virgin (or not so local in times of scarcity) would be pegged down on the ice as dolly, towards which men of the glen, clutching their stones, would launch themselves flat out across the frozen ground. Only the winner scored, losers suffering the pain and indignity of having their rocks kicked away.

Rules
Depends on whether you go European or Canadian, playing the 3- or 4-Rock FGZ Rule . . . Either way, the object of the game is to score in

the house, having somewhere along the way earned the right to put the boot in your opponents' stones and knock them into oblivion. All must be done in accord with the Spirit of Curling: polite smiles and pleasant handshakes throughout (smirks permitted in some parts of Europe).

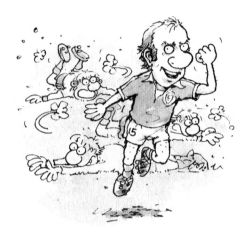

SEX·GODS OF SCOTLAND:
ARCHIE GEMMILL SCORES
FOR SCOTLAND
(Argentina, 1978)

STICK-AND-BALL GAMES

CURLING IS NOT the only sport in Scotland with a long history. Golf (first played by St Andrew) was much enjoyed by Mary, Queen of Scots, though she was never allowed into the clubhouse at Muirfield.

Shinty, *camanachd*, man-to-man golf with casualty lists, flourishes particularly in northern areas, which also play host in summer to the celebrated Highland Games. These are colourful occasions, in which kilted strongmen have the chance to show off their manhood in a variety of eye-watering challenges. Best-known of these is the caber toss, a feat of strength and cunning which takes years of practice to

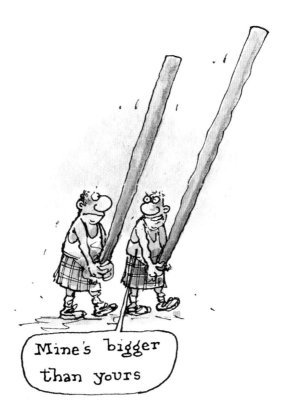

master. The first difficulty is in manipulating the slippery stick into position for action. Cabers come in different sizes: that used at Crieff is 17 ft 4ins long and weighs more than 150 lbs. Braemar's is longer but lighter, at 19 ft 9ins and 132 lb.

Other traditional sports (popular at Highland Games across the Atlantic) include sheath toss, fly-casting, speed drinking, throw-up, border collie, shortbread and bonniest knees competitions. September sees the annual World Stone-Skimming Championship take place at Easdale, attracting tossers from all over Europe.

11. Beastly Companions

I T'S A LONELY life up in the hills and the British have always had a fondness for animals. And that's as far as it goes. Anything more is an urban myth and a foul calumny on Celts, put about by smart-arsed Londoners fearful of rustics and savages roaming the wildernesses that stretch beyond the M25. That said, there are well-documented instances of shepherds entering into long-term loving relationships with members of their flock – and in the north-east, inflatable sheep are handed out to supporters of Aberdeen Football Club (The Red Army) to make up for disappointments on the field. According to Dr Ewen Bedde of the Centre for Ovine Relationships, sheep make difficult partners as, where one goes, the rest will follow.

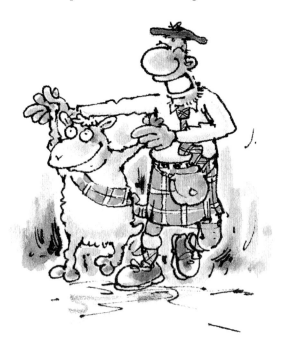

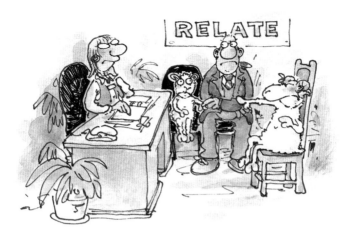

The good folk of Grantown-on-Spey
Make love in the time-honoured way,
In bed before sleep
With a favourite sheep
Or ram in the case of a gay.

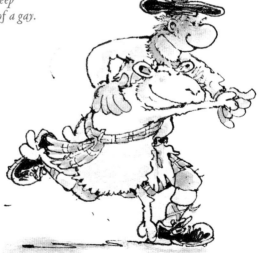

12. A to Z

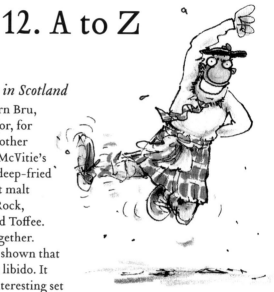

Aphrodisiacs

Ten Top Turn-Ons in Scotland

Loch Fyne oysters, Irn Bru, Scottish Blend Tea (or, for those that swing the other way, Camp Coffee), McVitie's Suggestive Biscuits, deep-fried Mars bar, Glensoddet malt whisky, Edinburgh Rock, McGowan's Highland Toffee. They work a treat together. Finally, research has shown that porridge does aid the libido. It must have been an interesting set of experiments that proved it.

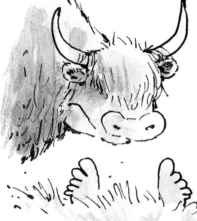

Pat on the Back

For cooling the ardour, try the close, warm breath of a Highland cow. As reported in *The Herald*, the Dutch town of Spaarnwoude recently brought in Highland cattle to graze a local nature reserve much frequented by open-air sex fiends. According to the mayor, 'the presence of the cows turns the people off having sex'. And it does rather add to the laundry.

Bondage

This is something that has really taken off in Scotland over the last thirty years and is now accepted as a regular part of Highland life. Companies all over Britain have come to recognise the value of sending their executive trainees and middle-management out into the wilds for a week or two of challenge, deprivation and corporate bondage. Survivors return to their desks weary, sore and unable to sit down, but older and wiser for the experience.

Contraception

It is impossible to get a thing on the radio apart from fizzing snitches of accordion music, interspersed with fish-prices from Peterhead and news in Norwegian, thanks to the distance from a transmitter mast and the close proximity of a large Cairngorm.

Cross-dressing

Practice confined mainly to royalty on the run or in extremis. Mary, Queen of Scots, fled Borthwick Castle in 1567 disguised as a man; Bonnie Prince Charlie escaped to Skye in the role of Betty Burke. In 1822 George IV came out in Edinburgh wearing pink silk tights beneath his kilt (see p. 24).

Cross-dressing has become more accepted in the twenty-first century. It is not uncommon these days to see a woman in a kilt, though usually more as a fashion statement than for purposes of sexual gratification.

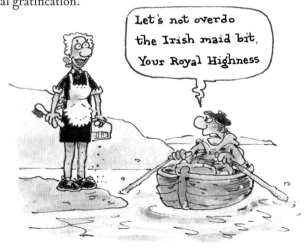

Deviation

Deviants, go elsewhere. Deviation is something that may well take place on the Continent (the French have arrowed road-signs pointing the way to appropriate venues), but it's not something that happens in Scotland, thank you.

Excitement

Discouraged on Lewis.

Exhibitionism

More famous for dourness and prudery (What's sex, please – we're Scottish?). Scots tend not to go in for public displays of affection, except at football matches. Flaunting oneself in a state of undress is something generally frowned upon, unless it's classical ballet. Alfresco grappling is not encouraged, as it upsets sheep and ramblers. Those so inclined should get in touch with the Fumblers' Association, whose members lay on regular outings. Having sex in the back of a car was never anything much boasted of in Scotland; this could be down to the long-standing popularity north of the border of the Scottish-built Hillman Imp.

Fetishism

Tendency to be overweight.

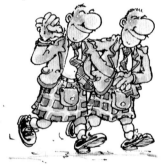

GAY GORDONS

Gay Gordons

Scotland has a long tradition of tut-tutting at unconventional relationships, as James VI discovered – firstly with regard to his cousin Esme, Duke of Lennox, and then with Patrick Gray (the one with rouged cheeks, scented gloves and twinkling earrings). These days, acceptance of such ways remains patchy, being confined to homogeneous zones around the big cities. Glasgow has a lively gay scene, with business folk quick to latch on to the importance of the Pink Poond. Here Same-Species Relationships are generally the norm and anything beyond that tends to be left to outlying parts of rural

Scotland. The Western Isles make up the one part of Britain to have banned 'geidh weddings'.

Group Sex

Or ceilidh, to use the proper term in Gaelic. Regular events, well advertised around the country, with no need for shyness on the part of any newcomer. Organisers are well used to catering for all types of occasion, from private function to large business dinner, and it is normal to provide a caller, armed with microphone/spotlight/megaphone and ready to instruct the nervous beginner as to which part of whose body should go where.

Heavy Petting

Close and intimate contact with large animal.

Infertility

Large parts of Scotland suffer from low fertility, thanks to rocky ground. Other parts make up for this, with more inviting terrain giving rise to general fecundity.

One of the techniques developed to combat fertility problems is that of in vitro fertilisation or the test-tube baby, as it is sometimes called. By this method, eggs are taken from the female and put in a test-tube for fertilisation by the male under laboratory conditions. This calls for some dexterity on the part of the male and caution in handling the test-tube.

Another technique, pioneered in Scotland with sheep, is that of cloning. Scotland is now overrun with identical-looking sheep.

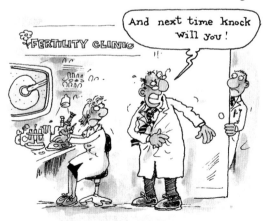

Jiggery-Pokery
Unfortunate consequences of unrestrained Scottish dancing.

Kissing
In all cultures, kissing comes in many forms, from the all-day, life-scarring wet snog to the nanosecond brief peck, followed by twenty minutes of disengaging earrings and bi-focals. In Scotland, too, there is every variety, from Ayr-kissing, cheek-swipes and deep throat excavation through to the full Glasgow Kiss needing stitches at the Infirmary. Gumshields a must.

Love
Deep relationship of heightened awareness, emotional depth, physical closeness and unconditional interdependence, involving feelings often unspoken, such as commonly exists between a man and his wallet.

Munro Bagging
Popular Scottish pastime of climbing up to above 3,000 ft and then removing your trousers. Competitive Munro Bagging: climbing up to above 3,000 ft and removing someone else's trousers.

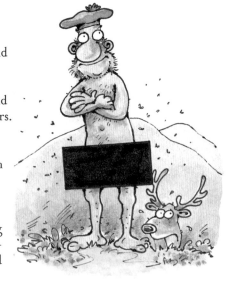

Nunro Bagging
Rare feat of de-trousering a nun above the 3,000 ft contour.

Nudism
Nudism has never been that big in Scotland for obvious reasons – the preachings of the Kirk and

the prickliness of the heather. And some of it could be climate-related, with local nudist organisations reporting a marked shrinkage of members in winter months.

In general, Scotland takes a relaxed attitude to nudism, providing ample opportunity in designated spaces run by Scottish Nature. In areas marked Reserve, naturism is encouraged but not compulsory. Do not stray unclad beyond marked areas. Spotted by a minister near Dingwall, the Naked Rambler was grabbed by the constabulary and detained at Wick.

Discretion is a virtue well prized in Scotland and the natural tendency north of the border, as with the Scotch egg, is to add a layer rather than to bare all. Most Scots prefer to keep their assets under wraps, especially when it's windy.

Over-age Sex

A bit of a sensitive issue, especially with younger people, over-age sex is something slowly on the rise in Scotland, thanks largely to the efforts of Grey Lib, 81–130 clubbers and the natural ageing of '60s rock-stars.

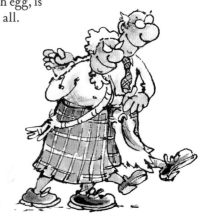

GREY GORDONS

Pipes

It was a brave soul who first discovered that a gentle nudge on the scrotum of a Highland bull would produce a plaintive moan at the other end. Braver still the person who found out that a prolonged squeeze could result in a series of different notes. And bravest of all the person who realised that said scrotum could be removed from the bull and blown through to provide more of the same music. Thus was the bagpipe born.

Of all the great experiences Scotland has to offer, what could be more romantic than a candlelit dinner, with piper on hand to serenade the love of your life with popular hits and tunes of your choice? Enjoy.

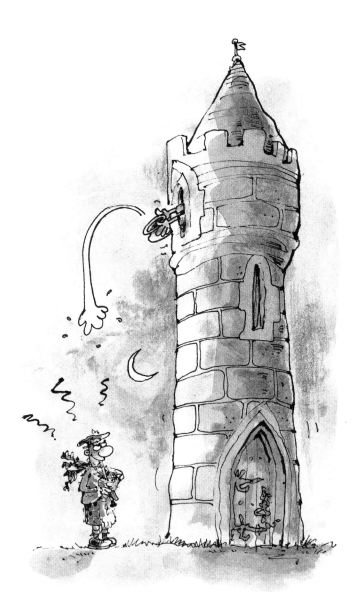

Quaich

Shallow, bowl-like drinking-cup, usually with two handles (not unlike a small chamber-pot in shape); traditionally passed round for the partaking of whisky; easily mistaken in the dark and the cause of much merriment.

Rugby Songs

'Four and twenty virgins came down from Inverness
And when the ball was over, there were four and twenty less'.

from *The Ball of Kirriemuir*: trad. Scottish ballad

The whole world over, sporting occasions are the traditional venue for celebrating in song great feats of local prowess. Scotland is no exception and *The Ball of Kirriemuir*, with its rousing chorus, is a firm favourite. What is now exciting cultural historians on both sides of the Atlantic is the quest to uncover the facts behind those exploits commemorated in song. In a joint venture of cross-disciplinary partnership, postgraduate students from Minnesota (Faculties of Hygiene, Leisure and Gender Awareness) have been working together on a research project which hopes to provide new insights into Scotland's rich and colourful past. One aspect of their work that has generated much interest is the Living History Re-enactment Project, which sets out to test the validity of claims put forward in many of the ballads under scrutiny.

Truth is often stranger than fiction. As was reported in *The Scotsman* of 9 June 2001, a group of twenty-four virgins from Inverness did contact London insurers Goodfellows in search of cover against immaculate conception before the millennium.

STD

Scotland's Health Service has long been recognised for its excellence in the treatment and prevention of transmittable diseases not for general discussion, viz. cold sores, kilt chafe, bluebag, sheep tick, goat pox, knee-tremble, caber itch, scab . . . Anyone so afflicted should hobble along to the nearest infirmary, where they can be assured of swift treatment, discreetly handled. Or seek friendly advice over the counter at any Rod & Tackle Shop.

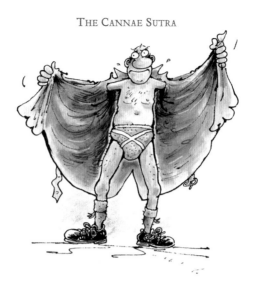

TV

TV stands for television in Scotland and has nothing to do with men in skirts. On 30 Oct 1925 Scotland's John Logie Baird, inventor of the Baird Undersock, demonstrated his new creation, built from a teachest, a hatbox, a biscuit tin, a darning needle, some sealing wax and a good deal of string. With this prototype, Baird produced some of the first fuzzy television pictures, showing a dummy's head in his London workshop. This set the pattern for decades of broadcasting to come.

Underwear

Never ask a Scotsman about his underwear. There's a risk he may just show it to you.

Venus and the Scotsman

Venus, Second Rock from the Sun that is, not Venus, the Roman Goddess of Love. The only feature on the planet Venus to be named after a person is the Maxwell Mountain Range, after Edinburgh-born James Clerk Maxwell. Physicist and all-round brain, Maxwell (1831- 79) did the sums to work out all the great advances of the last century, bar the ringtone. His prediction of the existence of electro-magnetic waves led on to X-ray, radio, radar, television and *EastEnders*; Maxwell's Equations opened the door to quantum physics and Einstein's Theory of Relativity. One hundred years before the Voyager probe could prove him right, Maxwell worked out what Saturn's rings were made of. And he was the man chiefly responsible for the world's first colour photograph. Lining up three magic lanterns to demonstrate the trichromatic process, Maxwell gave a bravura display of things to come. And the subject of this photograph – a raunchy nude maybe or a dazzling array of begonias? The man from Edinburgh (by now a Professor in Aberdeen) chose a piece of tartan ribbon.

Voyeurism
Use of long-range, high-resolution, night-vision binoculars, fast-focus stalker's telescope and similar optical and audio equipment in surroundings of Granton, Crathie and Bearsden. Common amongst Peeping Tams.

Waterbed
Not a good idea in the frozen north.

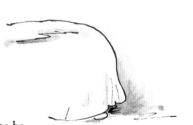

X-Rated
One of the first things trainee librarians learn is to seek out the famous f--ing scene in J.M. Barrie's children's classic, *Peter Pan*, and to set to with scissors, brown paper and paste. You all know how it goes. It's the one where they try it first on the floor and then from the beds – and find it quite heavenly.

Other titles from Scottish literature to be found on top shelves only:

Arthur Conan Doyle – *Round the Red Lamp*
Andrew Lang – *The Blue Fairy Book* (see also *The Yellow Fairy Book* and *The Violet Fairy Book*)
George MacDonald – *The Day Boy and the Night Girl*
Sir Walter Scott – *Death of the Laird's Jock*
Anon. – *The Lay of the Last Minstrel*

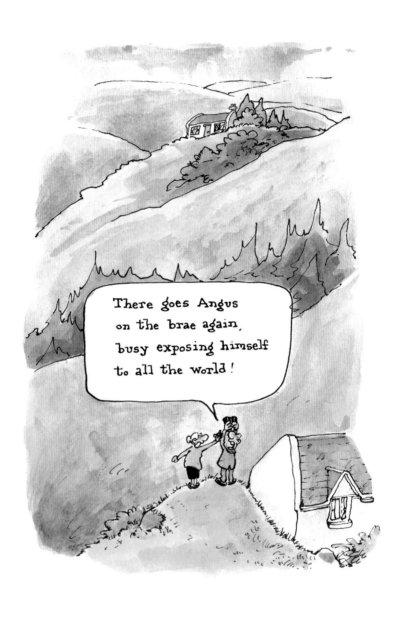

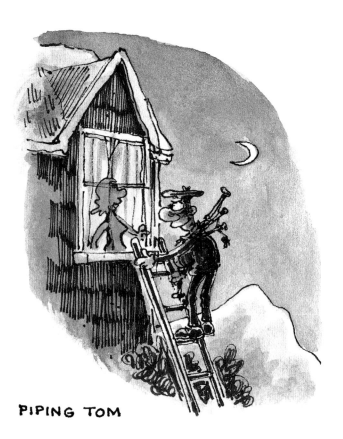

PIPING TOM

Yoof

Yoof knows it all and can't be told, except in matters of sex, of which yoof knows nothing, but still can't be told.

ZZZZZZ

The most active sound coming from a Scottish bed following intake of aphrodisiacs (see A above).

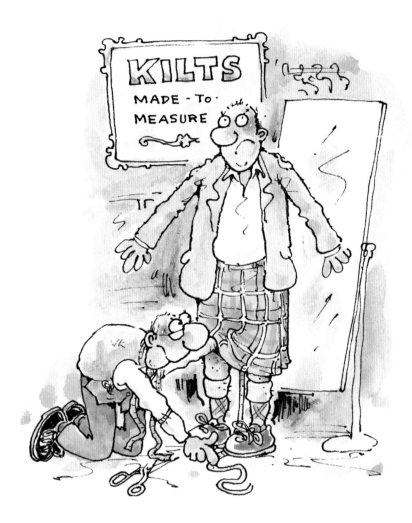

13. FAQs

What is worn under the kilt?
For Real Scots there is only one answer: the ghoolistra, traditional thong of plaited heather or broom, interesting for the different weave-patterns adopted by each clan and used for identifying bodies after battle or in the dark.

How far can I go?
In some parts further than others. Scots are proud of their right to roam.

How many sexually transmittable diseases can be carried by one dress-hire sporran?
As many as you like – there is no limit.

Why Bay City Rollers?
Why indeed.

Where do babies come from?
From supermarkets. You will have seen customers wheeling out babies on their trolleys along with other purchases.

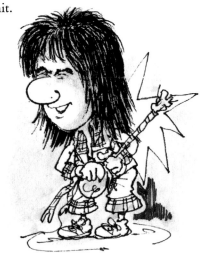

1970s SEX·GOD OF SCOTLAND: BAY CITY ROLLER

Is there an effective contraceptive for midges?
There is – particularly a morning-after pill – but problems remain in getting the little blighters ever to take the thing.

How do midges mate?
Most successfully.

That's no answer.
A little goes a long way.

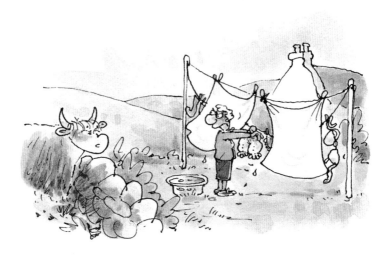

FURTHER AWKWARD QUESTIONS

If a golf-ball lands on a courting couple, how does that affect the scoring?

Do fish-farm escapees fight their way back into hatcheries to spawn?

Should auld acquaintance be forgot?

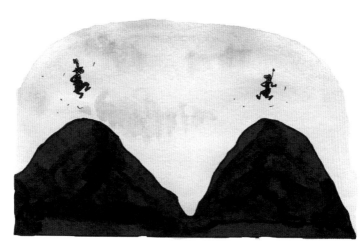

14. Words of Wisdom

SOME USEFUL SAYINGS

- Thrappled crawf hath muckle snit

- Tis mawkin's blooster that cantles the drouth

- Dinna graip the droddum of a dinsome howdie

- The last laverock hath twa ligs

- The whortleberry glypes its ain stane

- Aye, said the crocodile

A SLIGHTLY NAUGHTY SCOTTISH GRACE

May ye live as long as ye want to
And want to as long as ye live.

Trad.

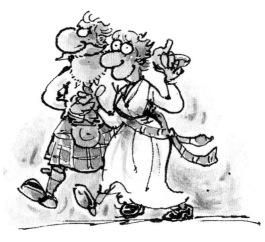

15. Fun Page

WORDSEARCH

Can you find the following words and phrases hidden in the grid below? Exactly.

sex, vice, perversion, unnatural acts, clootie dumpling, unnecessary behaviour

```
S C O T L A N D
C O T L A N D S
O T L A N D S C
T L A N D S C O
L A N D S C O T
A N D S C O T L
D S C O T L A N
```

WHERE THE . . . ?

Rearrange the letters to find the Scottish places:

NEVER SINS
DENUDE
CRY HOT LIP
BARE LADY
BOY TREMOR
FIRM NUDE LEN
RUDH BINGE
SAGG LOW
SORE LENGTH
O RAM BALL

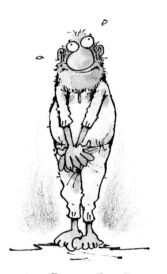

stark naked

Answers: Inverness, Dundee, Pitlochry, Aberlady, Tobermory, Dunfermline, Edinburgh, Glasgow, Glenrothes, Balmoral

114

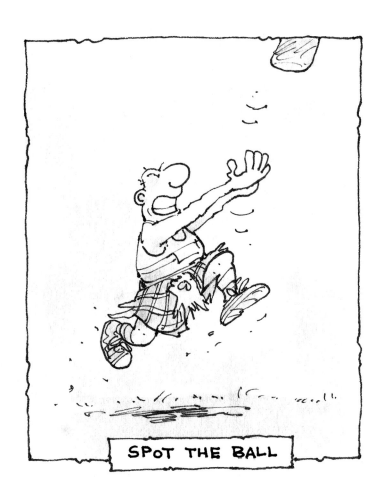

SPOT THE BALL

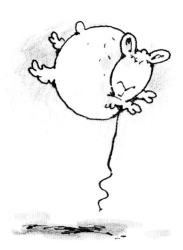

Inflatable Dolly

16. Glossary

alpha male – one just off an oil-rig

banff – slang for continuous stationery, documents, wastepaper; 'a load of banff'

bit of rough - extremely suggestive behaviour on the golf-course

bondage session – painfully bad S. Connery impersonation

cock-a-leekie – bladder trouble

cottaging – self-catering

Dick Institute – interesting local museum in Kilmarnock

dominie – traditional village authority-figure purveying sexual gratification with a whip

dounreay – fast breeder

droit de seigneur – getting laird

eightsome reel – wife-swapping

explicit – time to dive for the Off switch

extra-marital relations – too many in-laws

fernitickles – sensation created by walking through bracken in kilt

fochabers – mild expletive

foreplay – suggestive behaviour on the golf-course

gey – great, considerable (also, adv. rather, fairly)

heavy sex – anthracite

inflatable dolly – blow-up sheep

interruptus – get off at Paisley

kinky – from Kincardine

love triangle – three in a bed; Cameron, Finlay & Janet

monikie – salacious conduct with use of cigar

my ain folk – incest

nymphomaniac – one given to kissing on second acquaintance

orgasm – tiny sign of life, small creature with spelling difficulties

orogeny – mountain-building (geol.)

orogenous zone – Paps of Jura

pervert – person of artistic tendencies

perverts – two persons of one gender booking into the same hotel

sado-masochism – East Stirlingshire Supporters Club

setts – tartan patterns (see 'Joy of Sets')

sheep trials – series of local court cases best not gone into

smokehouse – place to retire to after sex

sporran – posing pouch

tosser – manipulator of caber

tongue – place in Sutherland

wick – place in Caithness

White Leather Club – traditional way of seeing in New Year in Scotland with a thong and a dance

FOR FURTHER READING

How to Have Better Sex (Jute Importers of Dundee, 1903)
Improve Your Sex Life: New Ways with Old Bags (Scottish Coal Board, 1924)
Intricacies of Sex (Jute Mills Co-operative, Dundee, 1948)

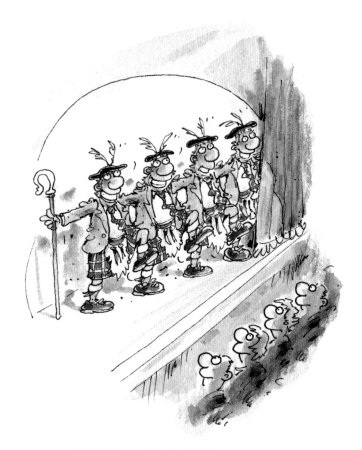

SATURDAY NIGHT SPECTACULAR
AT GLASGOW'S FAMOUS FOLIES BERGÈRES

Index

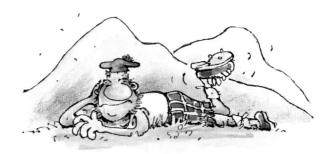